The Palgrave Lacan Series

Series editors

Calum Neill
School of Psychology and Sociology
Edinburgh Napier University
Edinburgh, UK

Derek Hook
Duquesne University
Pittsburgh, USA

Jacques Lacan is one of the most important and influential thinkers of the 20th century. The reach of this influence continues to grow as we settle into the 21st century, the resonance of Lacan's thought arguably only beginning now to be properly felt, both in terms of its application to clinical matters and in its application to a range of human activities and interests. The Palgrave Lacan Series is a book series for the best new writing in the Lacanian field, giving voice to the leading writers of a new generation of Lacanian thought. The series will comprise original monographs and thematic, multi-authored collections. The books in the series will explore aspects of Lacan's theory from new perspectives and with original insights. There will be books focused on particular areas of or issues in clinical work. There will be books focused on applying Lacanian theory to areas and issues beyond the clinic, to matters of society, politics, the arts and culture. Each book, whatever its particular concern, will work to expand our understanding of Lacan's theory and its value in the 21st century.

More information about this series at
http://www.palgrave.com/gp/series/15116

Gautam Basu Thakur
Jonathan Michael Dickstein
Editors

Lacan and the Nonhuman

palgrave
macmillan

Editors
Gautam Basu Thakur
Boise State University
Boise, ID, USA

Jonathan Michael Dickstein
Independent Scholar
Worcester, MA, USA

The Palgrave Lacan Series
ISBN 978-3-319-87644-3 ISBN 978-3-319-63817-1 (eBook)
DOI 10.1007/978-3-319-63817-1

Cover illustration: Deborah Ayers / EyeEm / gettyimages

Printed on acid-free paper

This Palgrave Macmillan imprint is published by Springer Nature
The registered company is Springer International Publishing AG
The registered company address is: Gewerbestrasse 11, 6330 Cham, Switzerland

Acknowledgment

We owe this collection to a series of conversations inspired by and between two conferences, namely, the 2016 American Comparative Literature Association Annual conference (specifically, the "Lacan and Philosophy" seminar) and the inaugural conference of LACK which took place a month later that same year. The hard work put in by all the contributors, the series editors, and the wonderful editorial and publishing staff at Palgrave Macmillan has brought it into its final form. Additionally, we thank Columbia University Press and *Cultural Critique* for allowing us to reprint respectively Jamieson Webster's and Kiarina Kordela's chapters. Lastly, we thank our friends and family for bearing with us through the process.

Contents

List of Figures

Chicken Knowledge: Or, What Does the Nonhuman Want?

Gautam Basu Thakur and Jonathan Michael Dickstein

One of the most striking recent developments in the humanities and the social sciences has been the shift of focus away from the human to the nonhuman. This shift is represented by not one but many concurrent critical and philosophical movements, concerning speculative considerations about topics such as ecology, post- and transhumanism(s), affect studies, systems and network theory, and object-oriented ontology. These considerations have led to, on the one hand, the exploration of the complex relational or congregational functions of nonhumans; and, on the other, the need to reimagine the world in the context of hyperadvancing technologies, swarming embodied communities, unending global conflicts, and looming specters of environmental crises.

Sometimes together referred to as 'non-anthropocentric humanities' or more colloquially as the 'nonhuman turn,' these new research directions

G. Basu Thakur (✉)
Boise State University, Boise, ID, USA

J.M. Dickstein
Independent Scholar, Worcester, MA, USA

G. Basu Thakur, J.M. Dickstein (eds.), *Lacan and the Nonhuman*,
The Palgrave Lacan Series, DOI 10.1007/978-3-319-63817-1_1

have proven vital to twenty-first century thought.[1] What though does this vitality entail? To begin to provide an answer, we might observe that each approach symptomatically stresses the problematization, critique, and rejection of human-only or human-centered approaches to a given object of study. Their common interest might be said to imply a characteristic rejection of what Immanuel Kant designated his Copernican Revolution—that is, a rejection of the replacement of the assumption that 'all our cognition must conform to the objects,' with the assumption that 'the objects must conform to our cognition.'[2] The result of such a rejection tends to amount to a decentering of the human in favor of a recentering of nonhumans and their world, thereby a vacating of the semblance of unadulterated anthropocentrism and a repurposing of the human–nonhuman dynamic according, not to conflict, but to symbiosis.

We are not claiming to dismiss this tendency outright—to reject the rejection of transcendental or even metaphysical idealism. We are claiming, however, that a purely (or overly) positive account of the original rejection proves too hasty. In this context, therefore, we posit the irreducibility of the Other insofar as the lack indicated by this irreducibility overlaps with the lack demonstrated by the subtraction of the subject from its world—that is, a subtraction leading to the subject being only a subject for its world but never a subject of it. Certainly, we grant the first thesis of any materialism: There is some One (i.e., a One that is materiality as such).[3] Nevertheless, as good dialecticians, we aim—even if in different ways—to privilege the necessary second thesis: Materiality is prior to thought.[4]

In this sense, we want to focus on what connects humanistic interest in the nonhuman with an eye more on what these interests lack than on what they possess. Specifically, the intent is to stress how the various strands of the nonhuman turn (with few rare exceptions) neglect the Freudian–Lacanian discovery of the (human) subject—that is, the subject whose desire is always and already the desire of the Other (the Other as not simply another human being but more importantly as the discursive system governing one's psychosocial existence). This neglect, we contend, often unfairly metonomizes Sigmund Freud and his disciplines as part of Western philosophy's bias toward the human, thereby a priori foreclosing any discussion along the lines facilitated by attention to the unconscious, favoring instead apprehensible or sentential facts about bodies, nature, and Humanity. Returning Freud and Lacan to the discussion of the nonhuman, we want to situate this book not on the side of nonhumans as such but rather at the gap, that is, the juncture between them and their subject.

Specifically, the goal is to initiate a much-needed constructive dialogue between theoretical assessments of Freudian–Lacanian psychoanalytic teachings and critical evaluations of nonhuman complexes and elements (e.g., material objects, uncanny things, climate, animals, the text, etc.)—a dialogue that repurposes the speculative directions for both. Without losing sight of the important epistemological and communitarian implications that the interest in the nonhuman has had in the context of twenty-first century scholarship, we ask therefore: How might—how must—Freudian–Lacanian teachings contribute to a constructive continued discussion? If nonhuman entails a relationship to its stem word (i.e., human) not according to inferiority, exclusive disjunction, or mere conflict, but rather according to its independence from, yet engagement with it, then the ambiguity of this term's semantic positioning with respect to its supposed opposite proves crucial for our book's intent and purpose. As such, individual chapters focus on exploring the nonhuman core of psychoanalysis and expanding on critical discussions of ecology, the animal, objects, and biotic and abiotic systems by means of Lacanian theory. To be precise, the aim of this collection is not to put the human back in the nonhuman, but rather to recognize the nonhuman that passes or poses as the human broadly conceived.

Freud, Lacan, and the Paradox of the Unconscious

Apropos the relation of psychoanalysis to nonhuman studies, the consensus tends to be on the side of sidelining, to wit excluding, Freud and Lacan from discussions of the latter. The common argument justifying this disregard pivots on overarching assumptions about and critiques of psychoanalysis's seemingly fixed (perhaps even outdated) focus on the human condition.[5] The problem, as critics might suggest, is then that

Freudian–Lacanian psychoanalysis is simply incompatible with the non-human turn.

We submit instead though that the problem has to do less with psychoanalysis itself and more with the hasty assessments of it. Indeed, to characterize psychoanalysis in terms of a strict genealogy of humanist thought is misleading. Introduced at the end of the nineteenth century, psychoanalysis shared with various previous schools (e.g., anatomical, geological, theological, philosophical, rhetorical, etc.) an interest in exploring humans' uncomfortable presence in nature.[6] In addition, like those thinkers before him, Freud directed his attention toward the border of the outside–inside division of the human and its Other. Unlike these thinkers, however, Freud did not deduce this division merely in passing from analysis to critique (i.e., Kant). Nor did he expose this division while charting the dialectical movement of becoming (i.e., Hegel).[7] Rather, Freud emphasized the border itself, the field in between, as what is really Other, thus seeking to articulate what this Other entails; he called it the 'unconscious' and determined its characteristics by way of analyses of its various effects in situations intersecting the then nascent fields of neurology, psychology, sociology, and anthropology.

For example, as early as the unpublished 'Project for a Scientific Psychology' (1895), Freud offered considerations concerning the *Nebenmensch* (neighbor) in terms of a distinct division between the familiar and what inhabits the familiar as its unknowable traumatic core.[8] Similarly, in later works, such as *Beyond the Pleasure Principle* (1920), in which Freud discusses the masterful play invented by his grandchild, the nonhuman environment of the infant's nursery—a wooden reel with string attached, the edge of the child's cot, a 'full-length mirror'—plays a crucial role in the child's conceptualization of identity in the absence of the mother. One needs to look closely at Freud's discussion of the child's game of 'disappearance and return' to realize the radical truth posited at the end of it: The human *always* appears after the object.[9]

About four decades later, Jacques Lacan intervened into this domain with the intention of rescuing psychoanalysis from its Anglo-American egotism by underlining this experience of the outside, which he considered crucial to the ground and trajectory of Freud's ideas.[10] Specifically, in 1936, he first presented his now well-known speculations about what he would call the 'mirror stage' of human maturation, during which an infant through a more or less automatic response to its reflection comes to develop the influential psychic functions for the negotiation of day-to-day observations and experiences (e.g., the ego, ego ideal, ideal ego, retroaction, identification, and desire). These speculations marked a distinct departure from theories privileging a healthy ego at the center of analysis by indicating how the 'I-function' requires external supports—in the case of the infant, a mirror, the *trotte-bébé*, and so on—and thus entails a constitutive misrecognition of its mastery over its own objective image.[11]

Lacan would reinforce and extend such conclusions throughout his career, articulating them in complex accounts of the registers of the psyche, their junctures, their abstract manifestations, and their concrete effects. Specifically, we might consider how these conclusions prove consequential in the now canonical Lacanian notion of the gaze and its partial basis in his tale of a youthful exchange he had with a fisherman (i.e., Petit-Jean) on the coast of Brittany. The exchange had to do with four key elements: a sardine can, its placement in nearby water (more generally in a spatiotemporal physical locality), a flicker of sunlight reflecting off its metallic surface, and a comment uttered by the (should we say valiant) representative of the working class: '*You see that can? Do you see it? Well, it doesn't see you!*'[12]

The elements of this exchange interestingly link 'matters of concern' close to the nonhuman turn—environmental pollution, the voice of rural subaltern communities, the agency of the thing, the ethics of the animal—to the psychoanalytic theory of the subject as suspended in the Other. Speaking to his students 40 years after the experience, Lacan referred to this anecdote to argue that what makes Petit-Jean's 'nonsensical' pronouncement significant has to do with the disquieting implications of being looked at in the moment of seeing something. When the human subject sees the Other, it also envisions itself in relation to the Other, such that there is already a picture from which it, the Subject, is absent. The emphasis here should be on the resultant paradox: The human grasps the nonhuman insofar as it grasps its relation to the nonhuman as part of the place that is Nonhuman—a place where this human subject was but now can only be lacking. Thus, much like the sardine can, the nonhuman (e.g., ecology, things, animals) proves to exist in a problematic nonrelation with the witness—the so-called human.

Chicken Knowledge (Is Dangerous!)

Slavoj Žižek often repeats a humorous parable that approximates some of the chief lessons to be taken away from such Freudian–Lacanian meditations on the unconscious vis-à-vis the human and the nonhuman. The parable begins with a patient at what should be called a psychiatric institution, who believes herself to be a single grain of wheat. When the treatment concludes, the patient's physician leads her to the exit to deliver a final farewell. The patient, however, pauses at the threshold with a disturbed expression. The doctor asks what the problem could be because the patient no longer believes herself to be a grain. The patient promptly replies: 'I know I am not a grain but does the chicken know that?'[13] As Žižek explains, this parable demonstrates how the unconscious operates from beyond: It is explicitly always already out there. Thus, to be a psychoanalyst means that one does not simply attend to internal (i.e., purely psychic) ailments but also to external ones. Moreover, and most important, psychoanalysis ought to bear on those seeming deviations at the border, the threshold, of the clinic, and the greater natural world.

Not too differently, as Richard Grusin notes in his Introduction to *The Nonhuman Turn* (2015), the field of nonhuman studies coalesces around the need to focus on 'animals, affectivity, bodies, organic and geospatial systems, materiality, [and] technologies' in order to examine how these directly and indirectly shape human lives and institutions.[14] Ewa Domanska also reiterates this point:

> [The k]ey research problems [in the field] include [questions about] the boundaries of species identity, the relations between the human and the nonhuman (human beings' affiliations with technology, the environment, animals, things), and questions of biopower, biopolitics, and biotechnology.[15]

More specifically, therefore, 'non-anthropocentric humanities' or nonhuman studies connect these diverse concerns with networks arranged by global capital, which should be 'understood as a force for exploiting and intensifying difference rather than as a tool for creating an equitable world,' and function to strategically determine what is properly human and what qualifies as nonhuman, or expendable.[16] '*Nonwhite, non-European,* and *non-Western* thus parallel the *nonhuman* and reveal what is at stake in using it.'[17] As such, the 'nonhuman' leads individuals to that singular ethical moment when we audit our role in the past and in the continuing destruction of the planet in close relation to local as well as global histories.

In this context we wager that Freudian–Lacanian psychoanalysis may serve as the chicken joke to the more serious odes to the nonhuman. One way of exploring this wager is through the question: Does the field of the nonhuman know how bound it is to the Symbolic, thus to the human? Inclusion of Freudian–Lacanian theory muddies the field, churning the muck to produce a new understanding of the human–nonhuman (non-) relation. The future of the field depends on it embracing the troublesome human. In the words of Donna Haraway, humans are not seen as 'a vanishing pivot between awful or edenic pasts and apocalyptic and salvific futures, but as mortal critters entwined in myriad unfinished configurations of places, times, matters, meanings.'[18]

We should clarify that *Lacan and the Nonhuman* does not simply endeavor to highlight the crass exclusion of the Freudian subject from nonhuman studies. Nor are we claiming that rehabilitating the 'human question' apropos Freud or Lacan will enact radical shifts to the main concerns of nonhuman studies. As convinced as we are about the usefulness of Freudian–Lacanian psychoanalytic theory for studying the nonhuman, we are equally aware of the need to examine nonhumans in Freud, Lacan, and psychoanalytic theory more generally. What truly energizes this book's content, therefore, is a long-pending dialogue between the various movements dubbed 'the nonhuman turn' and psychoanalytic theory.

Lacan and the Nonhuman

This book is divided into two basic parts, 'Definitions and Contexts' and 'Applications.' As a segment of the intended program to establish a dialogue between Lacanian theory and nonhuman philosophy, the chapters in the first part variously define the nonhuman in Lacan and Lacanian theory's engagement with the nonhuman.

In 'Toward a Less-Than-Human Psychoanalysis: Coitus Interruptus and the Object,' Jamieson Webster sets the tone for the anthology with an examination of the 'human' in psychoanalytic discourse. She begins with a simple rhetorical question: Is there a way to think about identity without referring to interiority—that is, does psychoanalysis allow something beyond subjectivity? She answers by revisiting Freud's theory of anxiety in the context of *coitus interruptus* and Lacan's subsequent underlining of the impossibility of recovering the subject except through certain relations with nonhuman objects.

Explorations of the nonhuman core of psychoanalysis or human-less psychoanalysis continue in 'A Horse: No Worse? Phobia and the Failure of Human Metaphors in Psychoanalysis' by Celeste Pietruzsa and Jessica Dunn. Focusing on clinical cases, this chapter claims that the phobic object plays a crucial role in the production of the subject. On the one hand, the human–nonhuman connection in phobia unravels a terrifying beyond of subjectivity, and, on the other, the phobic object opens the possibility for the analysand to creatively navigate sexual differences. Reading Freud's Little Hans case and Lacan's explication of it alongside two of their clinical cases, Pietruzsa and Dunn show the phobic object as responsible for revealing the deficiency of the human, its enduring myths, and the nonhumanness at the heart of the subject.

Kiarina Kordela's 'The Human Not in the Human' displaces the human further by claiming that it always comes after itself—that is, the human is already always posthuman. This displacement, she contends, is because of two central, concomitant processes that define modernity: (1) the development of the capitalist mode of production and (2) the secularization of thought. As for the belated self-consciousness of the posthuman character of humanity in the postmodern era of advanced global capitalism, she presents this as resulting from a general tardiness of consciousness that can grasp the structures and logic of its own conditions—in this case, capitalism and secularization—only once the latter's potential approximates, if not reaches, its fullest actualization. Kordela's repositioning of the human in the wake of the post-nonhuman proves invaluable for reexamination of another significant postmodern concept (i.e., biopolitics). She highlights biopolitical reappropriation of certain premodern Judeo-Christian concepts—specifically eternity, immortality, Jubilee, and sacrifice—, and the consequences of this reappropriation for understanding contemporary racism.

In '*L'extermination de tout Symbolisme des Cieux*: Reading the Lacanian *Letter* as Inhuman "Apparatus" and Its Implications for Ecological Thinking,' we find this revisionary urgency underwriting Kevin Spicer's assessment of the usefulness of Lacanian theory for contemporary ecological thinking. Noting that Lacan is summarily written off from discussions of the environment, Spicer contends that this unwarranted foreclosure serves only to obfuscate the nonhuman nature of reality, thereby rendering inconclusive 'current ecological philosophy's focus on the decentering of anthropocentric thought.' Observing the similarities and differences between Lacan's writings and recent scholarship on ecology, speculative realism, and object-oriented ontology, Spicer makes a provocative argument for understanding contemporary anxieties over the Anthropocene through Lacan's 'letter of the Real.'

Ed Pluth's chapter 'Lacanian Antihumanism and Freedom' continues reimagining Lacan in relation to the nonhuman by taking up the issue of freedom, especially the freedom attributed to machines by Lacan. He begins by noting that while Lacan spoke little about freedom, which he associated with humanism and sought to avoid, a careful reading of the Lacanian concept of 'full speech' however offers a radical antihumanist account of freedom. This antihumanism is best illustrated by Lacan's discussion of machines in his Seminar II as freer than animals. In this context, Pluth's chapter underscores just how full speech being machinic is truly free and the relation between this version of freedom in Lacan and Heidegger's concept of *Gelassenheit*.

In the manner of Pluth's discussion of Lacan with Heidegger, Paul Eisenstein's 'The Sovereign Signifier: Agamben and the Nonhuman' takes up Lacan alongside Agamben. Whereas Agamben's influence on the nonhuman turn is unquestionable, Eisenstein's pairing of Lacan with Agamben is a first. According to Eisenstein, Agamben's use of the neologism 'nonrelation' to capture the fractured biopolitical relationship between law and life resonates with and is better understood through Lacan's description of the Signifier as a stain forever separating humans from nature. He explicates this argument further by looking at lyric poetry in the book *Poems from Guantánamo: The Detainees Speak* (2007), especially the relationship between the primordial dislocation of the Signifier and the 'event of language.'

Eisenstein's chapter is a crucial component on the way to reassessing Lacan's position in the current climate of nonanthropocentric studies. A project seeking to initiate a Lacanian conversation with nonhuman philosophy must be aware of the risks incipient to it—chiefly, the danger of claiming provenance of the nonhuman turn solely in Freud's discovery. Eisenstein neatly complements the course of this book, as well as the chapters that come before his, by acting as a critical check against any hasty identification of Freud or Lacan as the originators of the nonhuman turn. As the final chapter in the first part, 'Definitions and Contexts,' it also establishes context for the book's second part, 'Applications,' which is concerned with the question of how nonreaders relate to texts; as Jane Bennett remarks, the latter are 'special bodies' responsible for making human perception about the planet more acute.[19]

The second part begins with Donald Kunze's 'Triplicity in Spencer-Brown, Lacan, and Poe.' He discusses the 'spooky coincidences' that connect Lacan's Real, George Spencer-Brown's Calculus, and the 'chiastic mirroring' in Edgar Allen Poe's short story 'The Purloined Letter.' According to Kunze, all three thinkers are Freudian kins: They 'combine "binary" investigations with an "orthogonal" excursion into issues that link the unconscious with *automaton*.' This kinship, he argues, brings them closer to the Freudian unconscious that exists without time, contradiction, and negation—a subjectless object. With this argument, Kunze hopes that OOO (or, Object Oriented Ontology) will also gradually acknowledge the importance of Freud's discovery in their continuing pursuit of objects without subjects.

Following such observations, Todd McGowan's 'Like an Animal: A Simile Instead of a Subject' develops the application of Lacanian teachings in nonhuman studies through a close analysis of animal metaphors. As McGowan explains, figurative phrases implicating various nonhumans or animals, such as 'dirty as pigs' or 'fat as a whale,' are habitually summoned for describing human extremes even though they often and paradoxically do not apply to the same creatures to which they refer.

Indeed, pigs are one of the cleanest animals, and even though whale's can have 50% body fat (in this sense, 'fat as a whale' is an accurate, if unflattering, simile), they cannot suffer from obesity. Thus, McGowan claims, invocations of animal metaphors indicate the subject's attempt to obscure the distortion that marks the conditions of its subjectivization. McGowan grounds this claim through an interpretation of the use of animal imagery in William Shakespeare's *Othello*, noting that these nonhuman representatives for the eponymous character function not only to dehumanize the Moor but also to negotiate the excess of his subjectivity.

In 'Beckett's "Marionette Theater": Psychoanalysis, Ontological Violence, and the Language of Desubjectification in *Stories* and *The Unnamable*,' Amanda Duncan continues the exploration of human–animal/nonhuman relationships through a discussion of Samuel Beckett's rejection of the humanist model of language, in which the capacity for speech is used to distinguish the human from the animal. Using the Lacanian premise of human alienation in speech, Duncan shows that in Beckett's novels, *Malone Dies, Molly*, and *The Unnamable*, this predicament is illustrated exactly where the textual production of meaning is staged as a form of ontological violence that reduces the subject to the passive silence of the animal, or to the nonhuman 'thing.' Beckett's writings present a paradox in which a 'life' is projected into and played out in language at the very point where the human 'disappears' into the Lacanian Real.

Calum Neill's 'Do Electric Sheep Dream of Androids: On the Place of Fantasy in Consideration of the Nonhuman' takes up for discussion a crucial related point: 'Can the difference between the human and the nonhuman be brought down to a question of belief?' Using the examples of human and replicants from Ridley Scott's film *Blade Runner*—Roy Batty (knows and believes he is nonhuman), Rachel (knows but does not believe she is nonhuman), and Deckard (neither knows nor believes that he is nonhuman)—Neill ponders the role of fantasy in grounding belief, arranging knowledge, and positing subjectivity in opposition to radical alterity.

Autonomous sensory meridian response (ASMR) videos from YouTube, the focus of Hugh Manon's 'ASMR Mania, Trigger-Chasing, and the Anxiety of Digital Repletion,' serve as a timely means to reflect on the implications of these themes in terms of new media. In the videos, performers 'speak directly into the camera, very close, in sibilant whispers, consonant repetitions, and with an attitude of oversolicitous caregiving,' producing in viewers either indefinable pleasurable reactions or complete disgust. The popularity of this 'media phenomenon' among millennials, Manon argues, emerges not from the promise of a lack of lack—someone is taking care of the viewer and/or listener—but rather because the videos themselves reinstate lack in an oversaturated digital culture.

Building on this theme, Jonathan Michael Dickstein's 'For the Love of Nonhumanity: Anxiety, the Phallus, Transference, and Algorithmic Criticism' punctuates the second part and the book by returning to the topic of Lacan's analysis of Poe's 'The Purloined Letter' to consider the cybernetic elements undergirding this analysis in terms of recent digital humanistic calls for rule-based approaches to textual interpretation. He argues that these approaches may prove viable if they are able to distinguish, measure, and take into account their potential to produce anxiety. Nonetheless, Dickstein suggests that our ability to appreciate this viability has everything to do with our proclivity to (mis)recognize the (counter)transferential relation in which these nonhuman structures situate us.

In sum, by engaging with the nonhuman turn, this book is also engaging actively with the death of the humanities. It would be naive to ignore how the recent interest in the nonhuman has coincided with and, to some extent, been impelled by the explicit devastation of the disciplines of the liberal arts—from the real effects of budgetary cuts to the symbolic ruptures of infrastructural upendings to the imaginary suturings of the fuzzy traditionalism of what, with Alain Badiou, we might call the late capitalistic logic of democratic materialism.[20] The present moment thus behooves us to embrace the incredulous—that which is beyond the pleasure principle, what Freud called the death-drive and Lacan the Real qua impossible. In this moment, we may confront the knot that is our nonhumanity and perhaps—albeit rarely—come to embrace the courage to cut it.

Notes

1. Ewa Domanska 'Beyond Anthropocentrism in Historical Studies,' *Historein*. 10 (2012), pp. 118–130; p. 118. Richard Grusin (ed.), *The Nonhuman Turn* (Minneapolis/London: University of Minnesota Press, 2015).
2. Immanuel Kant, *Critique of Pure Reason*, trans. Paul Guyer and Allen Wood (Cambridge, UK: Cambridge University Press, 1998), p. 110.
3. Compare Jacques Lacan, 'May 17, 1972,' from Séminaire XIX: … Ou pire (Unpublished, 1971/1972) and Lacan, *Book XX:* Encore (1972–1973), trans. Bruce Fink (New York: W. W. Norton, 1998), p. 5. Cf. also Alain Badiou, 'Lacan: L'antiphilosophie 3' (1994–1995), notes Aimé Thiault, transcription Francois Duvert, http://www.entretemps.asso.fr/Badiou/94-95.htm. Accessed 1 Dec 2016.
4. Badiou, *Theory of the Subject (1982)*, trans. Bruno Bosteels (New York: Continuum, 2009), p. 193.
5. See, Derrida *The Animal Therefore I Am* (New York: Fordham University Press, 2008); Agamben *The Open* (Stanford: Stanford University Press, 2004).
6. To an extent, the Freudian science has its roots in the rise of modern science, the Renaissance of the arts, the reformation of religion, the expansion of the mercantile middle class, the formal doctrine of the nation state, and the age of revolution and its aftermath. Its broad genealogy might be traced from prehistoric mythology and Greek tragedy to sixteenth-century humanist texts, anatomical writings, and Shakespearean theatre to eighteenth-century psychology/moral therapy, German Idealism, and, even, Romanticism. Supposedly, Freud himself credited the poets—Sophocles, Shakespeare, and Dostoevsky—for 'discovering' the Unconscious, relegating his contribution to formalizing the discovery. See https://www.freud.org.uk/about/faq/ (accessed 31 Mar 2017).
7. See Kant (1998); and G.W.F. Hegel, *Science of Logic*, trans. George di Giovanni (New York: Cambridge University Press, 2010).
8. Freud, Project for a Scientific Psychology (1895 [1950]), trans. James Strachey, Complete Psychological Works of Sigmund Freud, Vol. I (London: Hogarth Press, 1966), pp. 331.
9. Freud 'Beyond the Pleasure Principle' (1920). *The Standard Edition of the Complete Psychological Works of Sigmund Freud, Vol. XVIII*, trans. J. Strachey, 24 vols. (London: Hogarth Press, 1955), pp. 3–64; 15*n1*.

10. See, for example, 'Phallic Phase and the Subjective Import of the Castration Complex' in *Feminine Sexuality: Jacques Lacan and the École Freudienne*, J. Mitchell and J. Rose, eds., trans. J. Rose (New York: Norton/Pantehon Books, 1985), pp. 99–122, 106.
11. Lacan, 'The Mirror Stage as Formative of the *I*-Function' (1949), in *Complete Écrits* (1966), trans. B. Fink (New York/London: W. W. Norton, 2006), p. 75.
12. Lacan, *The Four Fundamental Concepts of Psychoanalysis*. Seminar Book XI (1973), trans. A. Sheridan (New York: Penguin, 1977), p. 95; emphasis in original.
13. Žižek, 'Notes Towards a Politics of Bartleby: The Ignorance of Chicken,' in *Comparative American Studies: An International Journal*, 4(4): 376–377.
14. Grusin (2015), p. vii.
15. Domanska (2012), p. 119.
16. Ursula K. Heise, 'Globality, Difference, and the International Turn in Ecocriticism,' *PMLA*, 128(3): 637, 2013. For more specific explication, see Richard Iveson, *Zoogenesis: Thinking Encounter with Animals* (London: Pavement Books, 2014). In *Zoogenesis*, Iveson follows Derrida to argue that the murderous exclusion of the animal sets the stage for similar exclusion of people deemed not human or less-than-human. This logic underwrites a large chunk of the nonhuman turn including postcolonial ecocriticism, ecofeminism, animal, and animality studies.
17. Marianne Devoken, 'Guest Column: Why Animals Now?' *PMLA*, 124(2) (2009), p. 363.
18. Donna Haraway, *Staying With the Trouble: Making Kin in the Chthulucene* (Durham/London: Duke University Press, 2016), p. 1.
19. Jane Bennett, 'Systems and Things,' in Grusin (2015), pp. 234–235.
20. As Badiou writes in *Logics of Worlds* in 2006, 'the crucial teaching bequeathed by Lacan remains the following: it is in vain that some, under the impulse of democratic materialism, wish to convince us, after the comedy of the soul, that our body is the proven place of the One. Against this animalistic reduction, let us repeat the Master's verdict: "the presupposition that there is somewhere a place of unity is well suited to suspend our assent."' Trans. Alberto Toscano (New York: Continuum, 2009), p. 482.

Bibliography

Agamben, Giorgio. 2004. *The Open*. Stanford: Stanford University Press.

Badiou, Alain. 1994–1995. Lacan: L'antiphilosophie 3. Notes Aimé Thiault. Transcription Francois Duvert. http://www.entretemps.asso.fr/Badiou/94-95.htm. Accessed 1 Dec 2016.

———. 2009a. *Logics of Worlds* (2006). Trans. A. Toscano. New York: Continuum.

———. 2009b. *Theory of the Subject* (1982). Trans. B. Bosteels. New York: Continuum.

Bennett, Jane. 2015. Systems and Things. In *The Nonhuman Turn*, ed. Richard Grusin, 234–235. Minneapolis/London: University of Minnesota Press.

Derrida, Jacques. 2008. *The Animal Therefore I Am*. New York: Fordham University Press.

Devoken, Marianne. 2009. Guest Column: Why Animals Now? *Publication of the Modern Languages Association* 124 (2): 361–369.

Domanska, Ewa. 2012. Beyond Anthropocentrism in Historical Studies. *Historein* 10: 118–130.

Freud, Sigmund. 1955. Beyond the Pleasure Principle (1920). In *The Standard Edition of the Complete Psychological Works of Sigmund Freud, Vol. XVIII*. Trans. J. Strachey, 24 vols. London: Hogarth Press.

———. 1966. *Project for a Scientific Psychology (1895 [1950]). Complete Psychological Works of Sigmund Freud, Vol. I*. Trans. J. Strachey. London: Hogarth Press.

Grusin, Richard, ed. 2015. *The Nonhuman Turn*. Minneapolis/London: University of Minnesota Press.

Haraway, Donna. 2016. *Staying With the Trouble: Making Kin in the Chthulucene*. Durham/London: Duke University Press.

Hegel, G.W.F. 2010. *Science of Logic*. Trans. G. di Giovanni. New York: Cambridge University Press.

Heise, Ursula K. 2013. Globality, Difference, and the International Turn in Ecocriticism. *Publication of the Modern Languages Association* 128 (3): 636–643.

Iveson, Richard. 2014. *Zoogenesis: Thinking Encounter With Animals*. London: Pavement Books.

Kant, Immanuel. 1998. *Critique of Pure Reason*. Trans. P. Guyer and Allen Wood. Cambridge, UK: Cambridge University Press.

Lacan, Jacques. 1971/1972. Unpublished, May 17, 1972, from Séminaire XIX: …Ou pire.

———. 1981. *The Seminar of Jacques Lacan, Book XI: The Four Fundamental Concepts of Psychoanalysis (1964).* Trans. A. Sheridan. New York: W. W. Norton.

———. 1985. Phallic Phase and the Subjective Import of the Castration Complex. In *Feminine Sexuality: Jacques Lacan and the École Freudienne*, J. Mitchell and J. Rose, eds. Trans. J. Rose. New York: Norton/Pantehon Books.

———. 1998. *The Seminar of Jacques Lacan, Book XX: Encore (1972–1973).* Trans. B. Fink. New York: W. W. Norton.

———. 2006. The Mirror Stage as Formative of the I Function (1949). In *Complete Écrits (1966).* Trans. B. Fink. New York/London: W. W. Norton.

Žižek, Slavoj. 2013. Notes Towards a Politics of Bartleby: The Ignorance of Chicken. *Comparative American Studies: An International Journal* 4 (4): 375–394.

Part I

Definitions and Contexts

Toward a Less-Than-Human Psychoanalysis: Coitus Interruptus and the Object

Jamieson Webster

Psychoanalysis has always traded on the figures of identity and interior depth. Even when these two are placed at odds with one another they are still bound in a tight embrace. I have become more and more wary, or weary, of both these figures. Is there a way of thinking of the subject without identity? Is there a way of thinking about the mind without reevoking, yet again, the trope of what is 'on the inside'? These questions seem to run head first into the wall of epistemological queries concerning what can be known, not simply about identity or the mind, but also how we place any knowledge or knowing in relation to them. It is not simply a question of how we know what we know about the mind, the body, and the self, but also how we envision what we think is known or supposed to be known and how. One might imagine that beginning to even ask these questions would have the most profound effect not simply on discourse

This essay is a version of a chapter from Jamieson Webster's forthcoming book *Conversion Disorder* (Columbia, 2018). We thank the editors of Jamieson's book, especially Yi Deng, for allowing us to publish it in our collection.

J. Webster (✉)
Eugene Lang College, The New School, New York, NY, USA

Psychoanalyst in Private Practice, New York, NY, USA

G. Basu Thakur, J.M. Dickstein (eds.), *Lacan and the Nonhuman*,
The Palgrave Lacan Series, DOI 10.1007/978-3-319-63817-1_2

but also in the actual consulting room of the psychoanalyst—how they conceive of what they are doing with patients. Is the analyst pursing the subject, even if it is Lacan's evanescent subject of the unconscious, or is it something beyond this?

Present-day psychology, neuroscience, and the empire of therapies trade on different visions of interiority, not only establishing a certain kind of doctor—so regal, so well informed, so clean—but also his or her object, which is often an identity to be consolidated, a depth to be plumbed and exposed, or a body that should be rendered seamless or declared out-of-order. I would like to find a different vision of psychoanalysis, or a different vision in psychoanalysis itself—one that finds a way to stop this machine and open into another territory. I imagine this as a territory that speaks of the drive more than it speaks about it, one that locates the limit of subjectivity in the direction of an outside.

Anxiety often is depicted by classical psychoanalysis and psychology as the affect of interiority par excellence, the signal of a certain humanization or existential quandary. Anxiety was distinguished from fear by appealing to an inside as the coordinates of identity. But, if one revisits the origin of Freud's theory of anxiety, it was not this 'inside' that mattered most, but a very strange 'outside'—what he would call *coitus interruptus,* which is how he explained the genesis of anxiety. Anxiety is an interruption of sexual enjoyment.

Lacan's reading of this psychoanalytic myth shows not the way back to a more secure subject, but a very particular relationship between a subject and nonhuman sexual objects. Lacan provides a rare and fascinating elucidation through one of his own cases, showing the importance of these concepts for a psychoanalytic cure. In this case, coitus interruptus and the object coalesce in a vision of a female sexuality that gives one a sublime map for a less-than-human psychoanalysis.

Coitus Interruptus

Of all the silly psychoanalytic ideas laid bare for all the world to see, perhaps none is as easily derided as the notion that 'anxiety' is a result of coitus interruptus—there, a terrible joke, along with Freud's other, early, childish theories of sexuality, such as the ones involving menstrual cycles and the nose. When it comes to anxiety in particular, Freud seems to need the link between neurotic angst and the nonhuman—albeit sometimes taking the form of biology, or some grain of the drive—to give substance to what is purely psychological, existential, and thus nebulous in the phenomena of anxiety. Yet, anxiety for Freud is a foolproof argument against any easy Darwininism, for it embodies an evolution gone haywire; the involuting effects of the civilizing function of society; and, simply, the sheer problem of sexuality. Anxiety alerts one to neurosis better than even the hysteric can, for at the very least, anxiety is something everyone knows about, whispered along back channels concerned with a delirious fear of an explosion of something unwanted or unwarranted, not on the inside, but always on the outside.

Orgasm, Freud tells us, is the ejection into the outside of the scraps or grains of libido, the exteriorization of the drive in bodily coitus. Anxiety, on the other hand, is these scraps trapped on the inside, unable to enter the stream of thought, or to simply return to the body, caught between here and nowhere. One can begin to see why coitus interruptus was an intriguing proposition for Freud. Something has been cut off mid-stream. Anxiety, both body and not body at once, or perhaps better, inhabiting the thin line between the two, must speak to some impossible process taking place between a body and the world, my body and yours. The theory is an unwitting early nod to the intersubjective matrix of the mind.

So, while Freud was developing the earliest threads of his theory of the pleasure principle, the question of anxiety and orgasm hovered in the background, tied to a deep hope of Freud for etiological explanations—coitus interruptus—that are also a diagnosis of culture. Let us turn this 'around' on Freud. The whole sexual apparatus of anxiety is seemingly not anxiety about sex or because of sex, but instead is the conflictual, tightly bound relationship between sexuality and anxiety. Freud makes anxiety a half-enjoyed interruption, the stoppage of orgasm, the characterological choice of this anxious pain against the pain of uninterrupted enjoyment—fulfillment as it might be called, with a degree of irony.

Anxiety is the choice to reinternalize the drive against its most absolute form of externalization, orgasm or conception. In this configuration, the perverse relationship to anxiety seemingly triumphs over the neurotic one to the extent that the perverse choice will always be to put it out there, on the outside—to act it out. The 'pervert' externalizes anxiety by making it belong exclusively to the other person, by making him or her anxious about sex, unveiling an anxious desire, while maintaining oneself at a remove. The 'neurotic,' on the other hand, stands still, refusing to confront the outside, screening out any involvement with the other, or making them simply an object of hate or repugnance. If the drive must be crystallized externally, but not in a perverse manner, in the form of what object would this take?

Anxiety is not a question of the delineation of something absolutely on the inside, but a question of how to place something on the outside. What is inside, what is outside, what is in between the two is not easy to distinguish, and anxiety alerts one to the problem. If we read Freud's correspondence with Fliess and his early musings on coitus interruptus and anxiety, he focuses quickly on what he calls the 'alienation' experienced between the somatic and the psychical, which, at this early point, is embodied by the choice of protection against conception, or hesitation around the repercussions of intercourse and the inability to find what he calls adequate satisfaction in a secure relationship. It is not clear what he means by this, especially 'a secure relationship,' but ultimately, the point is that the patient appears to choose a half pleasure to no pleasure or full pleasure. This half choice erodes one's somatic sexual constitution over time, leading Freud to a rather tense symptomatic loop—anxiety erupts because of interrupted pleasure and anxiety leads one to interrupt pleasure.

Masturbation becomes the hallmark of ruined libidinal potential, leading to a weakened constitution, weakened potency, which eventually becomes a disposition to anxiety, pessimism, and low self-confidence or, in other words, neurasthenia and actual neurosis. Freud even seems to react with surprise at a man who chose coitus interruptus when he seems to desire his wife and, at the time, only had two children; this man has 'coitus every 12–14 days or so; often, too, with long intervals. Admits that he feels limp and wretched after coitus with a condom; but not immediately afterwards, only two days later—or, as he puts it, he has noticed that two days later he gets digestive trouble. Why does he use a condom? "One should not have too many children!" ([He has] two.).'[1] I will not comment on the repetition of the signifier two, including coitus every two weeks. Freud seems bewildered that he would make a choice that goes against what would be an unencumbered pleasure, interrupting pleasure in a way that would always lead him to feel 'wretched.'

What is fascinating is that Freud's conclusions are invariably stacked against men. Males, Freud claims, are more likely to develop problems in the first decades of adult sexual life, women in the second (how ill-timed the sexes are). Why? In part because of masturbation, in part because of moral strictures, in part because of fear of infection and pregnancy, and last, the hint of a problem in relation to one's desire. Desire, so important to Freud's later theories, is hinted at in the case of a man, Herr K, who fell in love with a woman who was a flirt and experienced a 'great shock when he heard she was engaged to someone else. Now no longer in love—he attaches little importance to it—he went on.'[2] After his first intercourse with another woman he had an anxiety attack that night, and another a few days later. He uses a condom now, often feels limp after, and describes these interactions as forced. His libido has diminished over the last year.

In his discussion of this case, Freud links the diminishing libido to Herr K's 'hereditary disposition,' noting that 'his father suffers from melancholia...his sister has a typical anxiety neurosis.'[3] Nonetheless, Freud concludes that the 'enfeebled condition of sexuality' has its roots in 'the preparations for using a condom' insofar as these preparations 'are enough to make him feel that the whole act is something forced.'[4] The incident with the woman led to an increase in somatic excitation—something he attaches little importance to—which made a weakness in psychical mastery over somatic excitation apparent; or rather, it contributed to its more rapid degeneration, stressing an already weakened system. It was after this that the man decided to use condoms for fear of infection, what Freud says, laid the 'foundation for what I have described as the factor of alienation between the somatic and psychical.'[5]

The man, Freud says, 'brought psychical sexual weakness on himself by spoiling coitus for himself.'[6] Spoiling one's sexual life ultimately weakens the psychical and then the physical. At the end of the discussion, Freud was interested in Herr K's short attacks of melancholic mood, which he speculates must be of importance to anxiety neurosis because of alienation—but 'for the moment I can only make note of it.'[7]

What *is* important to note is how early on all of this is—1892. We are still eight years away from the publication of Freud's *The Interpretation of Dreams*. Yet, in this little case vignette, we can see that far from this being a description of 'actual neurosis,' it seems like a rather typical case of obsessional melancholia, replete with all the problems of rectifying the man's relation to his desire. He chooses to spoil coitus on every occasion, or to feel forced and persuaded, as if it was not his own pursuit. This bears a relationship to a choice and a pleasure experienced in the past that went awry—namely, his having been cuckolded—undoing that choice with every half decision, or half enjoyment, through coitus interruptus. This, for Freud, feels entirely masculine, and in fact he concludes on several occasions in his letters to Fliess that women seem to be less disposed to this version of neurasthenia—'normally girls are sound,' or they are only neurasthenic in the case of the inability to get pregnant, bad marriages with neurasthenic men, or around menopause.[8]

One ought to be careful when considering a woman's complaints around anxiety, Freud cautions; frequently, they are married to neurasthenic men who are making them hysterical. Besides, the more passionate a woman, the more she will react to the decrease in a man's potency, the vicissitudes of coitus interruptus, and fall ill. This he contrasts with anesthetic women or women with low libidos who could tolerate this situation more easily. Here we find a complete inversion between male and female reactions to coitus interruptus—passionless men cannot tolerate it, passionless women can, passionate women cannot, and passionate men can. Anxiety, Freud concludes, is in a close relation with sexual limitation. The more impudent and daring, the more one is likely to indulge sexually and thereby fend off neurotic illness and the vicissitudes of inhibition in the form of hesitation, self-protection, dissatisfaction, and even the kind of pessimistic melancholic mood that comes with the blows to confidence that neurasthenia exacts.

As Freud writes, '[i]n the absence of such a solution [innocuous methods of preventing conception and disease], society appears doomed to fall a victim to incurable neuroses, which reduce the enjoyment of life to a minimum, destroy the marriage relation and bring hereditary ruin to the whole coming generation.'[9] Coitus interruptus is destroying the family, to say nothing of a whole generation to come. Even, Freud tells us, 'the lower strata of society,' meaning the less civilized and so less neurotic, will succumb to it.[10] Neurasthenia is the future of civilization—a world of hesitant half orgasming men and more and more hysterical women. The end or truth of marriage as this hereditary ruin.

If the beginning half of *Civilization and Its Discontents* is concerned precisely with this intertwined relationship between pleasure and society, unpleasure and anxiety, the second half signals the changes wrought by Freud's second topology, which focuses on the problem of trauma, repetition, the superego, guilt, and aggression. But again, even with all his banging on about the death drive, Freud still sees the solution in psychoanalysis by being the ally of what pushes back against the costs wrought by civilization against desire. He imagines a civilization that could accommodate the something-unique in one's pleasure–unpleasure economy. These solutions are as equally on the outside as the original imagined solution of an innocuous method of preventing conception or disease, or what he comically prescribes as the easy and early access for young boys to good girls.

When looking at Freud's later, second topological model, he famously changes his theory of anxiety, making it the accomplice of the ego rather than of the libido and placing it before repression, not subsequent to it. Freud divides anxiety into two moments: In the first, anxiety is the result of trauma, or, the ego being overwhelmed by stimuli it was unable to prepare for or defend against; in the second, anxiety is a response to trauma, trying to master it, turn passive to active, by anticipating danger, sending out preparatory signals that take the form of anxiety. Fixation on the first moment is closer to actual neurosis, a system overwhelmed, while the second is psychoneurotic—a system caught in a kind of backlash. Small doses of anxiety are an attempt to preserve the status quo, to inoculate against further danger. Otherwise, the individual must turn away from the overexciting stimulus, away from reality, moving further inward. In both cases, we can see that repression is not operating all that well; this is why there is anxiety at the place where there ought to be *la belle indifférence* of the symptom. The symptom itself is a metabolization of trauma—a representative, or a strange kind of memory, within a psychic economy. The 'symptom' is a structure, and 'anxiety' is the devastation of structure.

Although this is certainly a twist in the tale of anxiety that Freud is weaving, he does eventually say that these changes are not really at odds with his original thesis. Libidinal tension makes the ego helpless, which is essentially how he defines both trauma and the concomitant response of signal anxiety. In both the original and the second model what is discharged as anxiety, he says, is *surplus* libido, and the economic implications are always the same—this surplus creates helplessness and anxiety. Rather than repression folding outside and inside together, with anxiety, everything becomes the internal problem of overstimulation, avoidance, and helplessness. Whereas this might seem disconcerting, like some degradation of the beautiful model of the mind in repression and symptom formation, there is something here that deserves attention.

Freud says that many have noted the relationship between anxiety and self-preservation, or anxiety and the fear of death, something that is certainly the wheelhouse of the ego. In these moments, he is fighting Rank's theory that anxiety comes from the trauma of birth, from the separation from the mother's body. He is quick to dismiss this equation because, he says, 'nothing resembling death can be experienced,' and if it is simply birth trauma, then why would not everyone be cripplingly anxious?[11] What we are witnessing with anxiety is a psychosexual, not an existential, problem.

What the ego does know, he claims, are losses and separations, especially those that hinge on psychosexual development. In fact, this is where we see anxiety in childhood, the first being separation anxiety or stranger anxiety in the infant once the representation of the mother has cohered enough so that the child can then imagine losing her. This occurs well after any supposed birth trauma and is linked less to the expulsion from the uterine environment and more to the nature of a representational mind and the consequences of pleasure. 'At birth,' writes Freud, 'no object existed and so no object could be missed.'[12] Repression mirrors the condition of being without an object, since the object, or object tie, is erased. With anxiety, on the other hand, the object tie is preserved but under the signal of apprehension concerning one's threatened attachment to it. The symptom is a return to objectlessness, or the symptom is a kind of psychical replacement for the anxious tie to the object.

In a moment I find rather surprising, Freud comes to reverse cause and effect entirely, saying that anxiety is not about the expectation of a danger, but the experience of and reaction to, a specific loss or separation, changing the emphasis from the imagined danger to the nature of the tie to the object. Here, Freud evokes an affective chain that begins with anxiety and is followed by helplessness, pain, mourning, and separation. He then wonders how he could have arrived at this conclusion because the reaction to loss and separation is pain and mourning, not anxiety. It is a question, Freud says, of undoing the ties that bind, or decathexis. Separation is an achievement at the opposite pole to anxiety and is related to the work accomplished by mourning that allows one to decathect a lost object.

It is here that we must return to the question of surplus libido discharged as anxiety, because regardless of whether one is experiencing curtailed enjoyment or the fear of libidinal satisfaction, whether the ego is overwhelmed by internal or external stimuli it cannot master, whether the system is going haywire and interpreting everything as a signal of danger, whether one is anticipating danger or fearing separation from a beloved pleasure, there is a surplus in relation to an object that is taking the form of anxiety. Freud here implies the necessity for a kind of working-over or working-through—perhaps in the form of a substitute object, perhaps in the form of a different satisfaction reached. Either way, what is being sought is the reduction of this excess of helplessness that is equivalent to whatever Freud means by separation, or even 'common human unhappiness.'

What we see in this tale of anxiety is something about the stakes of an analytic cure and the objects with which one must form a relationship. Freud's attempt to clarify the nature of anxiety leads him to consider what is distinct about the human relationship to objects, especially insofar as this tie is always sexual. In one sense, all modes of attachment to objects seem to be either pathologically anticipatory or retroactively symptomatic. A new relationship must be created. How can we live with less anxiety and more pleasure, or how does psychoanalysis convert one to the other? It is perhaps here that we might turn to Lacan who pushes both the question of pleasure and what the transformation of anxiety has to do with the end of analysis. For Lacan, anxiety emerges at the place where separation is a question—trying to draw out the thought concerning the decathexis of the object and the anxious reaction that can be provoked by this call.

If Freud folds anxiety into a developmental table—fear of the loss of the object, fear of the loss of the object's love, castration anxiety, or superego threats—Lacan reads these steps as the anxieties of being an object of the Other, a position that is certainly one the child undergoes. We are taken by others as a body, taken in by their enjoyment. Lacan transforms the question of the object into the question of being an object. Psychoanalysis is not concerned with a special human relationship to objects, like some moral tale of loving well, or cognizing the Other, but rather something more distinctly nonhuman or a relation to the nonhuman as such. Lacan shows that being the object can threaten the sense of separation integral to a sense of vitality. He sees in the series of lost objects (i.e., oral, anal, phallic, scopic, invocatory) a point of identification—to be sucked, shit, fucked, exposed, spoken. Here, there is a strange bidirectional movement: allowing oneself to be these things—why not, its enjoyable—and, on the other hand, breaking the absolute identification with the object. To be sucked or fucked is momentary, not absolute.

Through a consideration of this detachable, partial object that is enjoyed, the one highlighted by Freud in his theory of sexuality, Lacan locates a classic trope of hysteria. Specifically, Lacan refers to his arm, noting his ability to isolate and ponder it as 'the intermediary between my will and my act' and joking about how he might leave it in the subway or an analyst's office, like an umbrella.[13] This joke though is not only funny. What Lacan means to show with it is that anxiety, especially if it is castration anxiety, is not only about the question of dismemberment and bodily harm but is also the recognition of the unconscious in all this psychopathology of everyday life.

Lacan concludes that the fact of not controlling one's arm could be a point of assurance, because if I do not have it, then no one else does either. It is not a question of absolute control or self-mastery, or being out-of-control—a discourse every analyst will recognize immediately in the oscillation of patients' anxiety. All the platitudes concerning letting-go, including those steps involving giving oneself over to a higher power, file in. These are not wrong, as they never are. They simply miss, in their simplicity, what is more radical about the unconscious; here, in the specific nature of our relationship to repression and its coming acknowledgment in our anxiety-ridden life.

Anxiety arises in an in-between space in the sensation of sensing oneself as a body in relation to something outside, the sense of this foreign edge. Scratch the surface of anxiety and one will find an agoraphobia that eventually betrays a knowledge of the unconscious as it acts on the patient. Every action, when rooted in anxiety, is reduced to an act of controlling the appearance of this Otherness, either in oneself or the other person. Here we get a glimpse of why anxiety must be tied to sexuality. Regression for Lacan is regression away from the recognition of separation, calling up earlier phantasmatic modes of enjoyment, provoking the anxiety that wants to grind this sexual unconscious to a halt.

For Lacan, the meaning of separation is not, this is my arm and that is yours, my arm does what I want it too; it is instead, something more like, who knows whose arms any of these are, all the same, I'm doing just fine, it is not going to come off if my attention lapses. Separation happens despite the lack of any firm outlines rather than because of them. Lacan's reading of separation is not one that indulges in a definition of an individual sense of boundaries or achieved autonomy, but instead what it means to have a relationship with one's unconscious.

Lacan pushes this argument even further when he states that separation is most clear when it is an encounter with the lack of any common satisfaction whatsoever. It is at this point where anxiety erupts. This, he says, is made the most apparent in coitus interruptus, not as the failure to orgasm, but rather as the failure to achieve a common satisfaction that only further marks our separation. What is felt in the body as an interrupted enjoyment, the other's pulling out or pulling away before any conclusion is reached, is this sexual nonrelation. The illusion of 'commonality' cannot be reestablished. Lacan says that what we have with coitus interruptus is the bodily appearance of the fact of castration; this is why it is named as *the* source of anxiety by Freud. Lacan is concurring with psychoanalysis supposedly at its worst, uniting in his unique and paradoxical way, the early and late theory of Freud. 'Thanks to Freud, we have this cleaving point in our grasp. This in itself is miraculous.'[14]

It is not only the separation between sexual partners, but also what can be found is the separation that takes place at the hinge between the organ, most often the penis, and orgasm or ejaculation. One is stripped away when the other emerges—namely, by the fact of detumescence.

> I'll simply say that anxiety is promoted by Freud in its quintessential function right where the accompaniment to orgasmic build-up is precisely uncoupled from the engagement of the instrument. The subject may well be reaching ejaculation, but it is an ejaculation on the outside, and anxiety is provoked by the sidelining of the instrument in *jouissance*. Subjectivity is focalized in the falling-away of the phallus.[15]

This passage is fascinating for all the terms of separation that seem to constellate—from uncoupled, to sidelined, to falling away—around what Lacan will go on to name the 'deciduous' character of the object. Separation is not simply about the imaginary violence done to a mother's body, or the imaginary violence of the child's ejection from it, or even guilt about sexual enjoyment, but simply a fact of the individual, its separateness, that manages to escape our notice. Escapes, that is, except when we are anxious in the face of so much coitus interruptus.

Perhaps this helps one to understand why anxiety is the only real or true emotion for Lacan, this moment of facing a certain reality, being signaled to it. Besides, if one can make it to the other side of anxiety, then the rest of the emotions—always sexual, always so labile (e.g., love, hate, disgust, and ignorance)—can emerge in this changed economy of desire. Coitus interruptus and the theory of anxiety, then, is no joke. The figure of interruption, like the most powerful day residue found in incomplete acts, helps everyone to think desire and the body, materiality and language, together. It also opens the door to a nonphallic sexuality and a different configuration of anxiety and enjoyment.

It is important to note that these intimations around female sexuality are well before the conclusions supposedly wrought in the infamous later Seminar XX concerning *la langue* and surplus jouissance. In Lacan's reading of Freud's strange obsession with coitus interruptus, he sees not some silly overly biological redundancy, nor even some misguided sociological commentary, but this fascinating place where psyche takes form in an in-between: in between two bodies, in between the somatic and phantasmatic expectations aroused by a sexual relationship, in between anxiety and the symptom, in between inside and outside.

The overriding question for Lacan when it comes to anxiety is the relationship to the deciduous nonhuman object. The emphasis is on the object as objectal, as opposed to any idea of objectivity. The object drags one along, unconsciously, the autonomy of the subject increasingly abolished in this drift, contact with the nonhuman object increasingly rendering subjectivity less than human. At this edge, we might find a point of equilibrium or assurance, one that is decidedly without the subject, where inside and outside are established through what Lacan calls a 'circumcision' in the economy of desire. A separation must take place at the furthest and most foreign edge of ourselves, in contact with what is absolutely Other.

Lacan uses the surreal naturalistic fable of a certain kind of shrimp that needs to imbibe a grain of sand in order to establish equilibrium. The shrimp, he says, needs to take this outside inside. Nevertheless, it has to be the right grain of sand. Scientists have made them swallow all kinds of things that throw them off balance, including grains of metal that allowed them to play with the poor little shrimp using magnets. Strange that evolution can make room for something like this—like the shock of birth not as the separation from the mother's body, but this foreign exterior, oxygen, breath, invading from the outside. Separation, for Lacan, is an achievement, even when it is a fact, and this separation is always the separation of one's body from another's. It is up to psychoanalysis, he says, to do an exhaustive study of this frontier.

What is important here is so fundamentally counterintuitive, even counter to the sense we like to have of what Lacan goes on about. In this tale of anxiety there is very little about the metaphoric nature of the subject, nor even really the subject of desire. Instead, what we find is the syncope of the subject in an anxiety that finally pulls them to the edge of themselves. Women, Lacan goes on to claim, are much better at bearing this movement through anxiety. Men, especially when it comes to detumesence or castration anxiety, are in much worse shape. Freud marveled at the fact of how well women can live with frigidity, whereas for men, impotence often destroys them. Lacan himself seems to concur with Freud's conclusion arguing that women make better analysts in being able to tolerate anxiety.

Taking up the question of the end of analysis as a confrontation with castration, Lacan says that if one looks at the question of anxiety she or he might understand how analysis, after everything, ends up 'in this dead end whereby the negative that stamps the physiological function of copulation in the human being finds itself promoted to the level of the subject in the form of an irreducible lack.'[16] The confrontation with the bedrock refusal of castration is the key to ending analysis. Is this negative stamp of the physiological function of copulation on the level of the subject that surges up at the end of an analysis what Freud was after in naming coitus interruptus the source of anxiety? Is Lacan as ridiculous as Freud in these speculations?

Lacan's conclusions follow Freud: '[N]o desire can be fulfilled without castration. To the extent that *jouissance* is involved, that is that she has my Being in her sights, woman can only reach it by castrating me.'[17] He continues, mimicking Freud's despair by imputing it to his listeners: '[M]ay this not lead the male portion of my audience into any resignation with regard to the ever palpable effects of this basic truth in what is called, using a classificatory term, conjugal life.'[18] The effects on marriage are palpable, for both genders.

Lacan, however, carries on—at least for the women, how can we not see that when it comes to castration anxiety they are lacking nothing? She is already castrated, so to speak, and it is the other who has to bear its effects, which she would like very much because it would return her desire to her. 'The fact is that on this point she has nothing wanting' because she wants everything from the position that she holds, especially when she wants a penis.[19] In wanting this penis, perhaps, Lacan muses, what she wants is for the Other to be able to tolerate the castration implied in having a sexual relationship so that for once, her desire can meet with another's desire. This is Lacan's affirmative reading of female desire.

What the woman is, Lacan says, is somehow something more real and more true. None of this ultimately resolves the question of her desire, nor the question of her anxiety—she has trouble with it in her own right, including the feeling that what she has is not enough. Nonetheless, in the end, Lacan takes pains to say that her desire is not caught in lack in the same manner, and this margin gives her room in a fascinating way. Not having to bear the organ and the gap between it as instrument, deciduous object, and jouissance, Lacan can place her in another way in relation not only to what she is but also all that is. So much so, that the fact of wanting does not unravel her because taking an interest in the object, as an object of desire, entails far fewer, as he puts it, complications for her.

The object does not need to fill a lack in her; the object is additive, a surplus, like the grain of sand to the shrimp. Lacan insists that there is something truly original here. In saying it, he feels this is the only way to unravel something about the nature of penis envy that has haunted psychoanalysis as a deadlock since Freud wrote *Analysis Terminable and Interminable* in 1933. To elucidate this, Lacan goes on to provide a fascinating case, one of the few of his own that he spoke of in any detail. He begins:

> One day a woman tells me that her husband, whose insistences are, if I may, part and parcel of the foundation of the marriage, leaves her alone a little too long for her not to notice . . . This is when she comes out with a sentence . . . *small matter whether he desires me, provided he doesn't desire others.*[20]

Lacan notes that he will not say that this is commonplace—something about a woman's jealousy or possessiveness or whatever—but that we can only really understand it from the constellation of what follows, especially about the statement as a message from within the transference.

The withdrawal of the husband's insistences, an attention that sustains her and her complaint regarding his clumsiness, opens up a field of desire. Lacan says she begins to speak with particular precision about her state, 'bear[ing] witness to what occurs for her if, when she is driving, for example, an alert flashes up for a moving entity that makes her say to herself something along the lines of *God, a car!* Well, inexplicably, she notices the existence of a vaginal swelling.'[21] This woman's desirous gaze is returned to her through the withdrawal of her husband's. As Lacan puts it, 'any old object' can become the trigger for an experience of jouissance that arises like a flash, a signal, as the other face of anxiety.[22] The state, she goes on to say, stops of its own accord—it has a rhythm all its own that begins and ends by surprise.

For Lacan, this means that the analogy with the man—her tumescence—does not follow the same path—namely, from tumescence to detumescence. Rather, it transfers onto a whole field of objects, and then stops as abruptly as it started. The patient continues, following these observations toward Lacan, speaking to the peculiarities of the nature of their relationship:

> Each of her initiatives are dedicated to me. …I can't say devoted, she adds, that would mean it was done with a certain aim, but no, any old object forces me to evoke you as a witness, not even to have your approval of what I see, no, simply your gaze, and in saying that, I'm going slightly too far, let's say that this gaze helps me to make each thing assume meaning.[23]

What we see is that this object that enters into her sight and evokes a feeling of vaginal excitement is linked in some way to the function of the gaze in the transference that renders, as witness, what she sees as meaningful.

This is not the demanding clumsy gaze of her husband, nor even her desirous looking, especially looking for Lacan's approval, but something about the analyst as witness, the one who can be evoked as watching this emergence of desire in a field that surrounds her. This object can be any old thing, but in this there is a pivot between assumed meaning (or the object as desired by the Other for its place or meaning in relation to *her* desire, this specified aim) and jouissance. This is the circuit that the other is used to supporting. All of this is prefaced by a separation, a fact (her husband's leaving her alone a little too long) that sets off the session and this series of confessions.

Lacan carries on with his description of the session. She has an association to Steve Passeur's play *Je vivrai un grand amour* that leads her to speak about falling in love with her husband, and then to her first love. She says about this first love that she stitched a series of lies like a cocoon that she enveloped herself in—in order to be exactly what she wanted to be in his eyes. This gesture is not exactly one done for his gaze, but rather to support her own in relation to a first love:

> She comes back to the threading, still stitch by stitch, of this dedicating of each gesture, which is not necessarily a gesture supposed to please me, nor one that would necessarily be in conformity with my thinking. You can't say she was forcing her talent [for lying].[24]

She does not make herself into what he wants to see, but what she wants to see about herself through him. She needs him in this little game of love to become her own ideal image. What she does with Lacan is very different, which he notes:

> [W]hat she wanted was not so much for me to look at her as for my gaze to replace hers. *I appeal to the assistance of your person. The gaze, my gaze, is insufficient when it comes to capturing everything that stands to be absorbed from the outside. It's not about watching me do something, it's about doing it for me.*[25]

I find this moment absolutely beautiful, this idea of an appeal for assistance in order to capture the everything that can be taken in from the outside. The insufficiency of one when it comes to the desire for this absorption. It is not the strategy of first love where the other, this fiction, allows her to exist, but something else. The relationship with Lacan is another iteration on the question of the gaze, but this time she finds support through another allowing her to see the everything that is there for the taking. She is not taking the other in, duping him as it were, nor is she taken in by her own ideal; rather, she allows her gaze to drop by replacing it with the analyst's eyes, and it is through this falling away of the gaze that the world flares up—*God, a car!*

There is a funny question of *who goes too far* that circulates between Lacan and this patient in the attempt to characterize their relationship; both seem to return the question to one another again and again, trying to find the right angle. Lacan characterizes her desire saying that it is not about his looking at her—certainly it is not—but rather that it is a matter of his gaze replacing hers. But 'replacement' is his word, and it is not quite replacement, as she says, but assistance, dedication, assumption, witnessing—calling on this other set of eyes in order to allow or frame this space where any object can be a source of desire, a great love to live, a literal swelling in her surroundings. Her eyes are returned to her at the moment where the object appears in its intensity, as a source of excitement, differentiated from an indifferent surround.

This witnessing provides a possible assumption of meaning through the Other—but, this meaning is just meaningfulness in and of itself, meaning that it is not and never will be any meaning specifically addressed to this other gaze, or what this other gaze is imputed to want. It is not approval, as she says, but simply an indication of herself as wanting in this sheer metonymy of objects. It causes these objects to flash across her screen with an almost simultaneous movement in her own body. This wanting seems to need, at bottom, another that can want in kind, that can hold this place—without either attaching themselves to anything in particular. Is this not the very essence of transference love? Especially transference love as work? Lacan does not say it, but it is there.

Any 'common satisfaction' is dependent on some realized separation—which begs the question of what is common? What we see in this case is that by dispensing or letting fall her gaze she calls on the analyst to make the object of her enjoyment appear. Is this the same deciduous object that is embodied negatively in the anxiety of coitus interruptus? Or, is the object transformed when it becomes not the sign of separation but the consequence of it? Lacan ends this clinical vignette, or at least his direct account of it, contesting her use of the term 'remote controlled' with a political analogy:

I'm only isolating this formula because you may have read it in the papers in connection with that left-wing politician who…thought he ought to give us the immortal example of how, in politics, the left is always effectively remote-controlled by the right.[26]

I am not entirely convinced that she exercises such poor taste in her choice of words—after all, the distance between the screen and the remote feels right, or the remote as a double to a function already contained in the device it controls, to say nothing of the additive object that this remote is in itself. Nevertheless, what Lacan is at pains to argue on behalf of his patient is that what she is speaking about is not about any reciprocity or reciprocal relationship (e.g., the symbiotic system of a two-party political system). It is something else. The transference is not the establishment of reciprocity but the possibility that arises from the achievement of separation, an asymmetry that lends itself to the support that the patient can find in the analyst.

'So, where is all this leading us? To the vessel. Is the female vessel empty or full? It matters not because it is sufficient unto itself, even if it is to be *consummated stupidly*, as my patient puts it.'[27] Lacan returns to the idea that for the female, nothing is lacking, nothing is wanting. What this means is that the object does not fill in for a lack, nor is it desired on the basis of some lack—the supposed penis envy—but rather, that it is a surplus: 'the presence of the object is an extra.'[28] Why? Because, Lacan says, it is not bound to the 'lack of the object cause of desire, to the $(-\varphi)$ to which it is bound in men.'[29] Men have anxiety, he says, about not being able and women are something that fills in for what is missing—thus, the woman as phallus for the man. But then, he says, what matters here is 'to grasp the woman's bond to the infinite possibilities or rather indeterminate possibilities of desire in the field that stretches out around her'—namely, this everything that stands to be absorbed from the outside (Ibid.).

Infinite and indeterminate—this is a truth about the nonhuman or less-than-human object as sexual for Freud, something that Lacan here links to female sexuality in particular. Her anxiety, he says, is only the anxiety faced with the desire of the Other, and, at the end of the day, who knows what this Other covers over—Lacan will not engage in a quest for origins. In any case, the past matters little if she can awaken this object through the Other, her analyst, for her pleasure. 'She tempts herself by tempting the Other' and, as the famous story goes, she can tempt with just about anything; 'it so happens that this apple was already good enough, little fish that it was, to hook the angler. The desire of the Other is what interests her' in so far as it can come to support any old thing, any little fish or apple.[30]

For the man, on the other hand, things are the other way around—desire is a cover for anxiety, and jouissance is sustained in a close relation to anxiety, something that leads to all kinds of complications from idealization and debasement in the sphere of love, to the half pleasures of interruption, spoiling, and feeling forced. Desire and jouissance pull against one another at this hinge of anxiety with little room for transformation. Here, Lacan says, 'you can see the margin he still has to cover to be in range of *jouissance*'—as if he can barely find this edge, or evoke this object through the Other, make of it something at a distance from himself.[31] The woman is often soldered to him, like Lacan's patient's pestering husband. In addition, there is always something of an imposture in the realm of male desire, meaning that he is posing, wrapping himself, like our patient with her first love, in a cocoon, a fictional envelope—one often made from the fibers of the woman who he claims for himself.

Letting desire be seen from within these wrappings is often a source of massive anxiety, a moment of unveiling. For the woman, on the other hand, the question of letting it be seen is precisely what is played with. In fact for Lacan's patient this is where she finds her greatest pleasures:

> For women, whose danger at the very most comes from the masquerade, the something that is there to be let seen is what there is. Of course, if there's not much, it's anxiety provoking, but it's still what there is, whereas for men, letting their desire be seen essentially amounts to letting what there is not, be seen.[32]

This moment in the seminar is fascinating. Not only is desire a question of any object whatsoever, this infinite surplus relationship to the object world, but beyond that it hinges on a relationship of what there is, not what there is not. This 'what there is' is in an intransitive relationship to the Other, making oneself seen, heard, sucked, and so on, through temptation—using them to extract these precious nothings, these objects that open one's access to an infinite field of pleasure, if not love. It merely means having to let what is there reveal itself, to know the worth of crossing the threshold of anxiety—something indispensable for psychoanalysis. It is not a question of the object as what is lacking or lost, but simply revealing what is there and allowing the object to become this additive enjoyment, this surplus pleasure.

If psychoanalysis has tended to emphasize the internal world, subjectivity, and lack or loss, here Lacan reverses this almost entirely. He concludes this section of his seminar by addressing the men:

[S]o, you see, don't believe that this situation, whose demonstration might strike you as fairly complex, is for all that to be taken as something especially desperate. Though it most certainly doesn't represent it as something easy, can you fail to spot the access to jouissance that it opens for the man?[33]Lacan is suddenly less pessimistic than Freud, or even the recurring contemporary image of himself announcing the absence of the sexual relationship. Here, he shows that somewhere (i.e., on the side of the object), we can see the point of access. Lacan will go on to call on the psychoanalysts for an exhaustive catalogue of the frontier where anxiety meets with the possible appearance of the object—what he calls the cut-off point where the deciduous nature of the object reveals itself. Crossing this threshold may mean being able to reconfigure anxiety and pleasure in new ways, something he points to much later when he talks about the *sinthome*.

If the subject can reorganize something fundamental in relation to his or her own body, a potential writing or rewriting of the body, this is certainly something he says that we can see in the language of the circumcision of heart in Christian theology, when people say, *I want your heart and nothing more*:

> But, here as always, language betrays the truth....In the formula, I want your heart...as in any metaphor of an organ, the heart is to be taken to the letter. It functions as a part of the body, as, if I may say, part of the innards.[34]

The anxiety that comes with being the object of this desire must be seen as literal, read to the letter: *I want your heart*. I want your organ. I want to be the organ of your enjoyment. Desire, Lacan reminds everyone, is always the desire for a body. The problem here is that these bodies, or organs, will always be utterly separate—a desiring machine without a subject. 'If what is most me lies on the outside, not because I projected it there but because it was cut off from me,' he writes, 'the paths I shall take to retrieve it afford[s] an altogether different variety.'[35] The consequences for psychoanalysis seem vast, appear to compose an altogether different system and map than what typically transpires as its most basic coordinates.

Is it really then a question of psychoanalysis as a passage to the outside, an object-oriented psychoanalysis, that jettisons any idea of 'interior' life and even the coordinates of subjectivity, especially insofar as they rely on this inwardness? In the case of Lacan's patient in particular, we see a strange functionality arising between them like two bodies humming, a woman without eyes, an analyst without a body, and a nonhuman object given all the life there is to give between the two parties, this unveiling so that something flashes up before her eyes, from him to her and back again. The world is suddenly an infinite meaningful field without it, for all that, taking on any specific narrative. That was the problem with first love, with the traps of a fiction in which she wrapped herself. This gaze dropped, handing herself over to her indeterminate analyst's eyes, opens an entire new realm. Then is this not what Lacan says a woman always has wanted—the whole world and nothing more?

Notes

1. Sigmund Freud, *The Complete Letters of Sigmund Freud to Wilhelm Fleiss*, trans. J. Masson (Cambridge: Harvard University Press, 1985), pp. 195–198.
2. Ibid.
3. Freud (1985), p. 197.
4. Ibid.
5. Ibid.
6. Ibid.
7. Ibid.
8. Ibid.
9. Freud (1985), p. 184.
10. Ibid.
11. Freud, 'Inhibitions, Symptoms, Anxiety' (1926). In *Complete Psychological Works of Sigmund Freud, Vol. XX*, trans. A. Strachey (London: Hogarth Press, 1959), p. 130.
12. Freud (1985), p. 203.
13. Jacques Lacan, *The Seminar of Jacques Lacan, Book X: Anxiety (1962–1963)*, trans. A. R. Price (Cambridge, UK: Polity, 2014): p. 217.
14. Ibid., p. 168.
15. Ibid.
16. Lacan (2014), p. 176.
17. Ibid., pp. 180–181.
18. Ibid.
19. Ibid.

20. Lacan (2014), pp. 187–188.
21. Ibid., p. 188.
22. Ibid.
23. Ibid.
24. Ibid.
25. Lacan (2014), pp. 188–189.
26. Ibid., p. 189.
27. Ibid.
28. Ibid.
29. Ibid.
30. Lacan (2014), p. 190.
31. Ibid.
32. Lacan (2014), p. 191.
33. Ibid.
34. Lacan (2014), p. 216.
35. Ibid., p. 223.

Bibliography

Freud, S. 1926. Inhibitions, Symptoms, Anxiety. In *Complete Psychological Works of Sigmund Freud, Vol. XX*. Trans. A. Strachey. London: Hogarth Press.

———. 1985. *The Complete Letters of Sigmund Freud to Wilhelm Fleiss.* Trans. J. Masson. Cambridge, MA: Harvard University Press.

Lacan, J. 2014. *The Seminar of Jacques Lacan, Book X: Anxiety (1962–1963).* Trans. A. R. Price. Cambridge, UK: Polity.

A Horse: No Worse? Phobia and the Failure of Human Metaphors in Psychoanalysis

Celeste Pietrusza and Jess Dunn

In Seminar VIII, Lacan describes phobia as 'the most radical form of neurosis.' Yet, compared to the number of case studies on obsessionality, hysteria, perversion, and even psychosis, there exists a relative paucity of Lacanian clinical writing on phobia. Although, from an Anglo-American perspective, this omission, practically, may be because of the fact that Lacan's major seminar on phobia—Seminar IV in *Book IV: The Object Relation*—has yet to be translated into English, this, we argue, is not enough to entirely account for phobia's glaring absence or, at best, cursory treatment in clinical writings by bilingual analysts. This chapter describes how phobias, in their connection to the role of the nonhuman or inanimate in the production of the subject, might point to a potentially terrifying beyond, of and for, psychoanalysis, at least of psychoanalysis as conceived of as 'faithful' to Freud or an anthropocentric interpretation of his works. In other words, how anxiety-provoking might

---

C. Pietrusza (✉) • J. Dunn
Department of Clinical Psychology, Duquesne University,
Pittsburgh, PA, USA

G. Basu Thakur, J.M. Dickstein (eds.), *Lacan and the Nonhuman*,
The Palgrave Lacan Series, DOI 10.1007/978-3-319-63817-1_3

it be, as analysts, to think that phobias, in their very existence and appearance qua solution, could be as radical, in some ways, as the psychoanalytic praxis itself?

Here, we discuss Freud's 1909 'Analysis of a Phobia in a Five-Year-Old Boy,' in which a young boy, whom Freud calls Little Hans, develops a phobia in which he fears the possibility of a horse 'biting him in the street' as well as a fear of 'horses falling down.' We discuss how Lacan, following Freud's acknowledgment that Little Hans's phobia was an 'elegant solution'[1] to Oedipal conflict and the problem of castration, articulates the operations of the signifier 'horse' to reveal the deficiency not only of the Oedipal but, perhaps, also the category of the human itself. We then present two case studies from our own clinical practices that illustrate how analysands' nonhuman phobic objects provided creative and flexible solutions to questions about Oedipal structure and sexual difference. Through these, we consider how phobias work to push psychoanalysis beyond itself into more unarticulated territories—in which a horse, for instance, does not symbolize but rather stands in for a father, a mother, a friend, a sister, anyone, anything…or, even, perhaps, nothing…else.

Widdling with the Nonhuman: Little Hans's 'Elegant Solution'

In the Little Hans case study, Freud uses detailed notes from the boy's father to construct an analysis of the development of his horse phobia. The case study also provided, for Freud, evidence and support for his own theories of infantile sexuality. Interestingly, Hans's parents both considered themselves followers of Freud and were looking to raise their son with minimal shame and intimidation around sexuality.[2] Freud himself met with Hans only once and, thus, many of what would be called 'interventions' in the case were actually spoken by Hans's psychoanalytically informed parents. Because a full exigesis of the case study is beyond the scope of this chapter, we focus here on three elements in Freud's writing that are important for Lacan's reading. First, Little Hans's interest in what he calls 'widdlers' (*wiwimachers* in the original German, the best equivalent in English to 'pee-pee' or 'pee-pee makers'); second, the incomplete castration threat made by Little Hans's mother; and, finally, the development and resolution of Little Hans's phobic symptom.

The notes of Hans's father begin from when Hans was just about three years old, as he developed an increasing interest in his 'widdler.' Hans began to inquire about what did or did not have a 'widdler' in the world around him. He asked his mother: Did *she* have a 'widdler'? His well-meaning mother replied affirmatively. He then asked about the presence of widdlers in animals and wondered whether a train had a widdler; then, only after this, asked his father if he had a widdler as well. Yes, animals have widdlers, his mother said; no, trains do not; yes, your father does. From these investigations, Freud noted, Hans was beginning to develop 'an essential characteristic for differentiating between animate and inanimate objects.'[3] In this interpretation of the function of Little Hans's widdler inquiries, however, we can see Freud's own anthropocentric assumptions concerning the importance and even the veracity of the categorical distinctions of human and animal, animate and inanimate in the psychic life of Little Hans. Freud cheekily notes that Little Hans seems to be a 'positive paragon of all the vices' in his polymorphous sexual interest in his mother, sister, and male and female peers of his own age, and yet he discounts the possibility that it might extend to trains and horses as well.

In *Anti-Oedipus*, Deleuze and Guatarri go so far as to credit Little Hans, the 'little Spinozist' and polymorphous pervert, with the insight that locomotives do in fact possess the mechanical equivalent of a 'pee-pee maker': the smokestack of the train is a protrusion that expels toxins from the body of it in the form of smoke just as the human protrusion does so in the form of urine.[4] Approached in this way, we already can begin to anticipate the radicality of Little Hans's position, even prior to his confrontation with what Lacan calls the 'sexual difference' between men and women.

During the same developmental period of Hans's fascination with widdlers, he also was confronted with an ostensible castration threat from his mother, who, when she caught him touching his penis, said to him: 'If you do that, I shall send for Dr. A. to cut off your widdler. And then what'll you widdle with?'[5] Although Freud argues that this threat would later have an effect on Hans's psychic life, at the time the boy was unfazed and told his mother that he would widdle 'with [his] bottom.'[6] As such, the castration threat did not affect, at that point, his psychosexual development or sexual behavior. It is only about a year later, after Hans's unsuccessful attempt to 'seduce' his mother into touching his widdler while she is powdering his genital area that his horse phobia emerges. Freud decisively notes that phobias and anxiety hysterias are '*par excellence* the neuroses of childhood' and, in many ways, normalizes Hans's anxiety, writing that it 'corresponded to repressed erotic longing [and] was, like every infantile anxiety, without an object to begin with; it was still anxiety and not yet fear.'[7] As such, Freud comes to understand Hans's anxiety as a longing for something forbidden that cannot be fully satisfied: his desire to sleep—or 'coax,' as Hans puts it—'with Mummy.'

Following this, Freud looks at how Hans's free-floating anxiety around his wish to 'coax with Mummy' ends up binding itself to another, different object: the horse in the street. This does not mean, Freud notes, that one should think of the horse as a substitute for Hans's mother. In Freud's meeting with Hans, he learns that Hans is particularly disturbed by the way horses look and 'the black around their mouths.'[8] When Freud asks for further elucidation, Hans clarifies it as 'the black round the mouth'—he means a moustache. As Hans's father also has such a moustache, Freud makes the interpretation to Hans that he is afraid of his father, as he fears he will be angry that Hans loves his mother so much.

Confirming this hypothesis, Hans's father later reports that his son's 'suppressed hostile wish is turned into anxiety *about* his father, and he comes in to me in the morning to see if I have gone away.'[9] Hans subsequently develops a new aspect of his phobia, in which he becomes afraid that 'horses will fall down,'[10] which Freud later interprets as both a fear of and wish for his father's death. Freud thus concludes that 'Hans was really a little Oedipus who wanted to have his father "out of the way," to get rid of him, so that he might be alone with his handsome mother and sleep with her.'[11]

Like Freud, Lacan in Seminar IV conceptualizes phobia as arising from the incompleteness of the castration threat and Hans's only partial separation from his mother. He employs a structuralist reading to describe these turns in the case study wherein the 'paternal function,' or father's prohibitory 'No!,' is not fully recognized by Hans; thus, what Lacan calls 'symbolic castration' is not entirely carried out.[12] Where Lacan diverges from Freud is in how he reads the paternal function as not equivalent or limited to the actions of the actual, living father. Lacan, instead, looks at how 'father' functions as a signifier—what he will instead call the 'Name-of-the-Father'—as what intervenes between the child and the mother's desire. Whereas the Name-of-the-Father might be linked, for some neurotics, to signifiers related to another person or institution related to the Law or Symbolic, in the case of Little Hans, a horse, instead, is raised to what Lacan calls the 'dignity' of this signifier.

Unlike in Freud's reading, the horse is not, for Lacan, a symbol *of* the father but rather makes up for the absence of the father and, as a substitute, operates 'as a *construction* that will allow the paternal metaphor to be set into place.'[13] Thus, the phobic object 'horse' works in the place of the father as an 'all-purpose signifier' to shore up the precariousness of the Name-of-the-Father and the paternal function. As such, for Lacan, it is not Hans's father, but rather, the phobic object 'horse' that allows Hans to make sense of sexual difference and therefore the Symbolic world.

From this, one can see how Lacan pushes the importance and role of the phobic object much further than Freud does. The horse, in its various manifestations (e.g., biting in the street, falling down with a cart), in Lacan's estimation, as a signifier, can stand in for any number of separate signifieds, which Hans is both drawn to as well as wishes to avoid because of the anxiety they provoke.[14] The horse qua phobic object thus operates as an 'empty signifier' that must serve as a way to organize and make sense of the real limits of the body and to stop, as Lacan writes, 'the whole signifying system [from] fall[ing] still further into nothingness.'[15] As Palomera notes, for Lacan, the phobia (i.e., Oedipus) is a myth used to resolve contradictions (e.g., the dilemma of sexual difference); however, it is, unlike Oedipus, a deeply personal and not universalizing one.[16]

Flame On!: Alex's Conflagration

As an example of the way in which a phobic object, in analysis, moves beyond a functional analogue of the paternal law, and instead supplants and surpasses it, we provide here, first, a case study from Jess Dunn's clinical practice. The client, whom we hereafter refer to under the pseudonym 'Alex,' presented with the fear of her house burning down as a result of 'faulty wiring,' a phobia she had harbored since early childhood. This case study investigates the processes through which nonhuman phobic objects intervene as a third between mother and child, thus interrupting and constraining the maternal dyad and providing a means through which Alex could begin to make sense of sexual difference.

When Alex, a Caucasian, lesbian-identified woman in her twenties, began therapy, she spoke first of her childhood home, which she shared primarily with her mother, from early age, when her parents divorced and Alex's father moved overseas, until Alex was 18. She described her relationship with her mother as a near-constant battle concerning Alex's (in) ability to adhere to expected gender roles. Alex's mother would purchase her 'gifts' that she deemed suitably feminine for her (e.g., dresses and stuffed animals in pastel hues). A particularly bitter site of battle was Alex's hair that her mother insisted remain long.

Although Alex reported constantly keeping alert for any signs of immigrant conflagration in the house, she never spoke of her fears to her mother, but instead was intermittently and privately vigilant. Her mother was a heavy smoker and Alex kept constantly on watch, especially when her mother was not present, for the smell of smoke. In therapy, she pointed to an electrical outlet and described an image that came to her of smoke pouring out of the outlet. When the therapist inquired further about this, she responded that it looked to her like cigarette smoke being exhaled, where the top two slits were nostrils and the round hole below and between the two slits, a mouth. Like Little Hans's association to the horse and the 'black round the mouth,' Alex saw a prohibitory face.

A parallel can be drawn here between Hans's horse falling down in the street and Alex's 'faulty wiring' and resultant electrical fire. Alex's fear of the house burning down thus also can be read as a wish, an ambivalent expression of hostility, hatred, and aggression. The phobia, which Alex did not articulate prior to therapy, thus, made space for the existence of a mother who was neither omniscient nor omnipotent, and the work of separation that distinguishes phobia from perversion or psychosis.

Alex next spoke in therapy about how, at the age of 18, she moved from her childhood home to live with friends, took a job as a line cook, and started wearing her hair cropped close to her scalp. When she began her first serious romantic relationship, however, she found herself in an antagonistic erotic relationship with another woman, whom we will call 'Marta.' As with her mother, Alex spent much of their relationship fighting. She struggled against Marta's criticisms of her appearance, which she called 'sloppy and immature,' as well as Marta's insistence that Alex not spend time with her female friends. So, again, Alex found herself in need of an intervening third.

A month or so before the end of their relationship Alex developed severe psoriasis on her calves, shins, and feet. She had never experienced any dermatological problems up to this point. Marta, however, had been suffering from psoriasis for some years. Alex often complained that her psoriasis did not so much itch as it 'burned' and that sometimes she would have to bathe her legs in cool water because they were 'on fire.' She also remarked that she thought the appearance of the rash looked like burns on her skin.

In this iteration the symptom moved from the environment to Alex's own body and yet continued to function in much the same way by both prohibiting and permitting desire for the (m)Other woman. The 'burning' rash intervened between Alex and her girlfriend both materially and psychically. The association of a physically painful burning sensation with contact between Alex and Marta can be seen here as a sort of psychic punishment or deterrent from continued contact with her. It also altered Alex's physical appearance, marking her body so that it was further removed from the kind of physical attractiveness that she thought Marta wanted. The symptom echoes the conscious resistance Alex employed against her mother's attempts to feminize her by cropping her hair.

Likewise, as in the case with the earlier phobic intervention, the symptom expressed her anger and hostility toward her girlfriend. In session, Alex would often say of Marta: '[S]he really burns me up.' This proclamation that her ex-girlfriend 'burns [her] up' also can be understood as an expression of arousal as well as anger. The burning rash then could be seen as the result of her passions becoming ignited, the torch she carries for Marta. As before, this burning ultimately extricated her from her overwhelming interlocutor while still allowing for the possibility of Alex's own desire.

Several months later, Alex's entrance into a new erotic dyad necessitated yet another iteration of the phobic symptom: The manifestation of the phobia closest to her childhood preoccupations and the one that finally brought her to treatment. Alex began dating a woman we will call 'Marney,' whom Alex often angrily described in sessions as 'clingy.' One night while sleeping in Marney's room, Alex detected a burning smell coming from the electric heater above their bed and, soon after, the room began to fill with smoke. Following this incident, Alex once again became preoccupied with the fear that an electrical fire would break out and did not return to Marney's apartment after this. Over the next year Alex's fear extended to ovens and electrical appliances at the restaurant where she worked. Alex stopped plugging in her cell phone and could only charge it by asking others, particularly Marney, to do it for her. Alex was no longer able to stay in her house, nor her bed.

As Alex's phobic objects became more varied and numerous, she became more dependent on Marney. When they were together, Alex was constantly asking her to 'plug it in.' In this request we see echoes of little Hans cheekily requesting that his mother powder his '*wiwimacher*.' By getting Marney to 'plug it in,' she was able to enjoy the erotic experience of watching a woman plugging in her power cord and unplugging the prongs from an electrical socket, a very material enactment of sexual difference, indeed.

Remarkably, this manifestation of her phobic symptoms intervened in more than one dyad at once. After Alex became fearful of the ovens and other appliances causing her to lose her job as a line cook, she moved back into her childhood home with her mother. After her return home, the symptoms Alex experienced as a child intensified, leading to arguments between them that often elevated to screaming fights and, in a few instances, nearly came to blows. The source of these fights often revolved around her mother's treatment of potentially flammable items or electrical appliances and/or her mother's dismissal of Alex's concerns. Alex described in great detail watching her mother pull the vacuum cleaner cord out of the wall from across the room, which 'bent the tines of the plug.' Her mother's violent unplugging of the power cord is in stark contrast to Marney's compliance with Alex's request to 'plug it in.' Whereas the latter shares a structural commonality with Little Hans's expression of his desire for his mother to touch his '*wiwimacher*,' the former is akin to his mother threatening to have his 'widdler' removed.

Alex responded to her mother's attempted (or failed?) castration of the electrical plug with rage that she described in session thus: 'I was, like, *flame on*!' Alex associated from this expression of rage to the 'Human Torch,' a character from the film and comic franchise *The Fantastic Four*, who cries 'flame on!' just prior to bursting into flames that neither extinguish nor consume him. As with Hans, who produced a solution of 'widdling with his bottom,' Alex produced through a cathexis with the phobic object the solution of becoming a human torch that is enflamed without being destroyed, whose fire is inextinguishable by others and yet can be ignited at will.

To make sense of the capacity of the phobia to intervene in both the maternal dyad and the dyad between Alex and her girlfriend, we must turn to the event that precipitated the onset of the phobic symptoms. Alex woke up in Marney's bed to the smell of smoke. When she jumped up and turned on the lights, she discovered that the electric heater anchored above their bed was 'smoking.' The smoking heater, in that moment, brought together, in its materiality, the prohibitive fear of being consumed by the flames of desire, the hostile wish to destroy, and the permission for Alex's desire for the 'smoking' mother–girlfriend. We can think here of Little Hans's longing for as well as prohibition against 'coaxing with Mummy.' This intersection of Alex's psychic arrangement and the material incident touched off a retroactive process in which the cathexes that had not been entirely addressed by the first manifestations of phobia began to shift.

As the associations and images began to exhaust themselves, Alex's symptoms began to wane. She broke up with Marney and had begun to speak in session of her fantasies about various women she worked with, whom she referred to as her 'work girlfriends.' She experienced fewer intrusive thoughts of her personal electronics sparking and starting fires in her mother's house and her place of work and, eventually, was able to plug them in and leave them unattended without concern. Her psoriasis started to ease and, at the time of her terminating sessions, was completely inactive. Just prior to her termination, Alex came into session and said she had been enraged that morning over an argument with her mother and remained so until starting her shift with one of her 'work girlfriends.' She described her anger thus: '[A] match that lights a line of gasoline that leads to a gasoline truck that catches on fire and explodes and it's parked at a gas station which explodes even more and pretty soon there is fire everywhere and nothing puts it out.' When the clinician repeated 'nothing puts it out,' Alex paused and responded with a smile: 'Well, women.'

What was remarkable about this case to the clinician was the way in which, as Freud remarked in the case of Little Hans, the patient, in many ways, seemed to analyze herself—or, perhaps, the phobic object and the patient along with it, shifted and adapted to each iteration and repetition of the structure. The phobic object thus accomplished the task of separation while preserving the client's desire and her enjoyment of sexuality: Little Hans can still 'widdle with his bottom.' We argue that the facileness of the phobic object, as raised to the dignity of the signifier of the Name-of-the Father, lies precisely in its nonhumanness. Even though the Name-of-the-Father is not, in itself, qua signifier, human, it all too often becomes conflated by patients and even analytically influenced therapists with its human referent.

The nonhuman, however, sidesteps what Deleuze and Guattari call '[t]he familialist reduction, in place of the drift of desire' and operates somewhere between metaphor and metonymy, thus never being fixed as either.[17] Without a human father and a human penis to constantly refer back to or maneuver around, the patient and analyst are freer in their associations and follow the ever-shifting 'drift of desire.' The 'smoking outlet' serves to animate Alex's forward-moving desire without necessary reference back to the human father, while still offering her entry into sexual difference, the limits of the body, and resolution of contradictions. Rather than shackling client and therapist to a structure that maps onto those of parents in terms of varying degrees of success or failure, the phobic object opens onto a loose and flexible assemblage in which there are multiplicities of positions, referents, and mobilizations of desire.

'Bugs' in the Room: Anjali's Infestation

In this second case study, we present a client from Celeste Pietrusza's clinical practice. In contrast to the case of Alex, who presented with a simple phobia, a young Indian-American woman who we will hereafter call 'Anjali,' presented for therapy with a vague and, at first, diffuse set of symptoms. In early meetings, she was highly anxious and said that she felt that 'everything was crashing down.' When she was asked to elaborate on this statement, she said that it was 'just a feeling' and that she 'wasn't sure what [she] meant.' In twice-weekly initial meetings, Anjali presented in a disjointed and almost disorganized fashion, jumping quickly and abruptly between topics, concerns, and even emotional states with few clear associations or through lines. At this time, Anjali had difficulty sleeping, had frequent panic attacks, and was plagued by an obsessive compulsion to organize and reorganize spaces—particularly closets and drawers both at home and work—according to various systems or schema. The only thing, Anjali said, that provided her relief from her constant anxiety, was cutting her skin in private with a knife, which she had done routinely, often daily, since middle school.

The clinician, in conjunction with her supervisor, a practicing Lacanian analyst, held open multiple possibilities for conceptualizing Anjali's case. Further analysis was to reveal that Anjali harbored a 'bug' phobia that could be said to, as Machado has observed in the course of development of a phobia, have been a way to 'put objects in place in order to organize the real.'[18] As such, Anjali's case, we believe, highlights the question raised in Lacanian clinical practice as to whether phobia—and its radicality—appears via symptom, structure, or both.

At the beginning of therapy, Anjali felt that her primary struggles circled around the ongoing arguments and negotiations over her parents' extended divorce proceedings. 'They've been fighting,' she said, 'for as long as I can remember.' Anjali's father, a first-generation Indian-American, and mother met for the first time when her mother arrived in the United States from India, for the occasion of their arranged marriage. Although Anjali knew that both her paternal and maternal grandparents came from Sikh families living in the same small Indian village, Anjali claimed she knew little else about her parents' marriage or relationship: 'I don't know the details, don't understand...and don't know if I ever want to.' This statement contradicted Anjali's descriptions of her relational patterns in most all other areas of her life: She often described herself as the 'messenger' and 'go-between' not only in her parents' divorce proceedings but also in dealings with other family members and even friend groups.

During her fifth session of therapy, Anjali reported her first dream. She described moving between rooms on different floors of her workplace. As she exited one of the rooms, she saw a woman she knew crying in the hallway and went to comfort her, but could not understand why she was crying. Anjali went upstairs into another room and began playing a video game. When she came out of this room, she saw an old friend petting his dog outside. When asked for her associations to this dream, she spoke explicitly to its doorways. Going into and out of rooms, she said, reminded her of her mother, whom in her childhood home, she said, would 'just stand in the doorway, watching me and my friends…spying on us.' Anjali said that the woman in the dream also made her think of her mother, who was diagnosed with borderline personality disorder and often suffered from what she called 'panic attack-seizures.' During these episodes, she would collapse on the kitchen floor and call for Anjali to 'cradle' her and 'caress [her] hair' until she calmed down or an ambulance arrived.

Anjali's symptoms and anxiety persisted in therapy until shortly after she related her next dream, approximately a month later. Anjali reported surprise at how 'realistic' she felt the dream was—during it, she said, she had not realized that she was sleeping and believed that it was 'actually happening' to her. Before going to bed, Anjali said she had seen a spider in her room, but 'lost it' and 'looked all over…but couldn't find it.' She reported feeling anxious as she tried to fall asleep: 'Maybe I swallowed the spider in my sleep? Do you think I swallowed it in my sleep? People swallow spiders in their sleep all the time, you know,' she said to me. She then went on to dream that 'the spider burrowed under [her] skin and began to lay eggs.' Anjali reported picking at her skin in the dream, described the sensation, and said that she was still 'itching' when she woke up.

From the dream, Anjali associated to a memory she had of another 'bug' that had 'found its way' into her dorm room: a centipede. The centipede, she said, had been 'crawling around all over' and 'kept getting lost…so I took a picture of it with my cell phone, so I would know where it was.' In this and subsequent sessions, Anjali spoke often and at length about both insects and other animals. She reported that she had a pet mouse, which would 'escape' from 'his' cage so often that she finally had to give 'him' away, and a hamster that kept getting 'lost in [her] dresser drawers.'[19] Anjali expressed that she 'hate[d]' when things were lost and, from this, spontaneously associated to her statement in our initial meeting that 'everything was crashing down.'

After Anjali's spider dream, sessions proceeded in a more associative, less staccato way. Anjali described both a fascination with and aversion to 'bugs' since childhood. When she was younger, she said she was often afraid of 'bugs in [her] room' and would be unable to fall asleep if she thought one was inside.[20] Anjali said she could never decide whether to 'squish' or 'save' insects and would spend considerable time ruminating without coming to any decision. Anjali connected her feelings about 'bugs' to her mother's family's Sikhism, a religion in which killing insects, she said, was strictly prohibited. Referring back to the centipede that was in her room, she said that since she had gotten a cell phone, that 'taking a picture of a bug' if she saw one was a way for her to manage her anxiety around it.

During this period of our work together, Anjali's symptoms subsided: She ceased cutting, her insomnia faded as she no longer spent late nights rearranging her room, and she reported only minimal anxiety without any panic attacks. Another turning point in therapy came approximately a year later, when, talking about a childhood trip to India, Anjali paused to mention that it was the only time she had been overseas. As her voice trailed off, the clinician asked, simply: 'The only time?' Anjali's eyes darted around the room quickly. 'There was this one other time…' she began, 'but I forgot about it until just right now.' She then proceeded to relate, in vivid detail, memories from a portion of a year she had spent in Dubai with her mother and younger sister at the age of five.

Anjali remembered leaving the United States suddenly in the middle of her kindergarten year, without explanation, while her father remained at home in rural Pennsylvania. Anjali described the tiny apartment ('only one room,' she said) in which she, her mother, and sister lived in Dubai. Among numerous other details, Anjali remembered a particular incident that happened right before they left that had 'confused' her: A man, Anjali recalled, seemed as if he was trying to break into their apartment. He demanded that Anjali's mother let him in, but she ran, grabbed scissors from the kitchen, put the chain lock on the door, and yelled at the man. Shortly afterward, Anjali returned to the United States, back home with her father, 'as if it had never happened.' Anjali remarked, aghast, that she could not believe that her family had never again spoken directly about this time in their lives.

Thinking back to fights between her parents as well as comments by them that had previously felt out of context, Anjali came to believe that her mother had planned to leave her father to be with the man who was later 'bugging' her in Dubai, and only returned to the United States because things had not worked out between them. After this point in therapy, Anjali reported little anxiety and, during the rest of time working together over the next two years, would present almost exclusively with stress-related depressive symptoms.

Although Anjali's bug phobia was not, as in the case of Little Hans or Alex, a simple phobia, the clinician considered, *après-coup* or after-the-fact, how it did, in many ways, serve as a structuring symptom for her analytic work. This is consistent with what Lacan, in Seminar IV, says about phobia as a way of providing an early origin or kind of proto-formation of psychic structure.[21] After working toward a resolution of her phobia in therapy, Anjali began to explore her own sense of gender identity and sexual orientation.

This follows what Ed Pluth, writing on Lacan's reading of Freud's case study, as Little Hans employing the horse phobia as a way to understand sexual difference and 'make sense' of what he calls 'sexuality "as such."'[22] A symptom (e.g., an animal phobia) Pluth argues, following Lacan, helps children take up the 'two enigmas' of both language and sexuality by 'forg[ing] a relationship between [them].'[23] Anjali, for instance, connected her memories of the 'bugging' incident in Dubai with the later emergence of her cutting symptom, as she recalled her first time cutting herself as a preteen with a knife during one of her parents' arguments. It was only after Anjali ceased cutting that she entered her first sexual relationship. The cutting was an auto-erotic type of experience for her that was done in private as a calming, relaxing activity; still, she also knew it was forbidden, taboo, and had told no one about until she came to therapy. In this light, Anjali's bug phobia can be seen as potentially negotiating the traumatic difference between her mother and her sexual partner: unknown lover as well as father.

For Anjali, her parents' sexuality and, following it, the details of their arranged marriage, were too anxiety-provoking to approach. Later in therapy, she would say that she feared and did not want to think that her birth had been the result of something traumatic (e.g., coercive or abusive behavior by her father). The signifier 'bug'—and the proliferation of bug and other phobias that were produced from it—could thus, through a kind of personal, cultural, and familial mythology, help Anjali at least temporarily to stave off the trauma of sexual difference.

Conclusions: Not One Horse, but Many

Phobia points to a radical and possibly terrifying beyond, of or for psychoanalysis in its junction with the inanimate and nonhuman. The phobic object does not metaphorically represent or stand in for a human absence, but rather creates a space for the failure of human metaphor. From a position of anthropic failure, the phobic patient cannot (re)solve the vicissitudes of the (m)Other's desire or the 'problem' of sexual difference through identification with a human father or mother or with the category of the human at all. In Freud's case study, he describes a game that Hans plays in which he bites his father, just as he feared the horse might bite him. Even though Freud reads this incident as Hans's successful identification with his father, if we understand the phobic object not as a representation of the father, but as Lacan does, as supplanting the father within the system of signification, we might consider that Hans instead is identifying with 'a bigger widdler'...or, worse, a horse. In their writing on Little Hans in *A Thousand Plateaus*, Deleuze and Guattari, pose the question: 'Is there an as yet assemblage that would be neither Hans's nor the horse's, but the becoming-horse of Hans?'[24]

As this chapter has shown through the two case studies, one can posit an answer in the affirmative. Alex engages in a becoming-flame with her ignition cry—*Flame on!*—that links her in a chain of associations to a character that is neither elemental nor human but something that occupies a liminal place in between. We can even imagine the ways in which Anjali engaged in a becoming-pest when she 'spied her' mother with her other lover. From a classically Freudian standpoint, there is something, indeed, horrifying about this proposition—the propensity and ability of children to create their own hybrid, proto-symbolic and nonhuman myths. Lacan, in his articulations of the operations of the signifier, sexual difference, and the Real, does not avoid this horror—the horror of the revelation of the deficiency of not only the Oedipal but also the human, itself.

Nonetheless, the greatest horror for psychoanalysis may not be in the failure of the human but the (re)productive 'success' of the nonhuman in phobia. Desire, for Lacan, is oriented toward any number of objects—phobic object, fetishes, or otherwise. In addition, while Freud utilizes the myth of Oedipus to understand the way Little Hans 'formalize[d] the impasse' of the Real of sexual difference, Lacan goes beyond, behind, or perhaps before Oedipus to look at the phobia as a proto-Oedipal production. Phobic objects, more than any other, have a tendency to proliferate—a phenomenon that behaviorists call generalization.

Unlike the *objet petit-a* in hysterical or obsessional neurosis, which constantly replaces one object with another in a chain of succession, the phobic object(s) are added to one another, populating psychic life with herds (i.e., swarms of objects that spread like wildfire). There is not, for Little Hans, simply a single horse phobia but rather many 'horses' in various states (e.g., biting or falling). Likewise, for Anjali, there was not a single 'bug' phobia, but many bug phobias: 'bugs,' in general, but also 'spiders,' 'centipedes,' and more. In the case of Alex, not only did her phobia accompany fire in several states (e.g., smoke sparks, flames, explosions) but also the nature of the object occurs in multiplicity to the point of being innumerable, for a fire is always already many flames.

As such, phobias can perhaps most radically reveal, in their materiality, the nonhumanness of sexuality and, truly, all of psychic life. Further, phobias in their multiplicity demonstrate the fallacy of the father, the phallus, even sexual difference between men and women writ large as too singular and centralizing to account for the complexities of polymorphous perversity (e.g., that of Little Hans). Instead, this creation of multiplicities points to the operations of sexual difference that can involve horses, trains, electrical outlets, smoke, spiders, and centipedes. Perhaps then, phobia has been avoided in some ways not because of the impossibility of treatment by means of psychoanalytic praxis, but the impossibilities of psychoanalytic theory to fully or adequately explain or represent this praxis. In other words, as clinicians, what should we think about the idea that we might only associate or, rather, do our own work of mythologizing about and around the connection between signifiers (e.g., horse, bug, what have you) and any number of signifieds?

Notes

1. Vincente Palomera, The Paternal Function and Little Hans' Phobia. *Newsletter of the Freudian Field* 6(1–2):49–61, 1992.
2. Sigmund Freud, Analysis of a Phobia in a Five-Year-Old Boy (1909). In *Sigmund Freud: Collected Papers, Vol. 3*, ed. E. Jones, trans. A. Strachey and J. Strachey (New York: Basic Books, 1953), p. 153.
3. Ibid.
4. Freud (1953), p. 256.
5. Ibid., p. 151.
6. Ibid., p. 152.
7. Ibid., pp. 257–168.
8. Ibid., p. 184.
9. Ibid., p. 187.
10. Ibid., p. 189.
11. Ibid., p. 253. As Hans's father notes at one point in his correspondence with Freud, as cited in the Little Hans case study, 'His fear of horses became transformed more and more into an obsession for looking at them. He said: "I have to look at horses, and then I'm frightened."'
12. Palomera (1992), pp. 49–61.
13. Ibid., p. 51.
14. Cf. Derek Hook and Calum Neill, Perspectives on 'Lacanian subjectivities,' *Subjectivity* 24(1): 247–255, 2008.
15. Jacques Lacan, Seminar VIII: Transference, p. 305; quoted in Bruce Fink, *A Clinical Introduction to Lacanian Psychoanalysis: Theory and Technique* (Cambridge: Harvard University Press, 1997), p. 163.
16. Palomera (1992), pp. 49–61.
17. Gilles Deleuze and Felix Guattari, *Anti-Oedipus: Capitalism and Schizophrenia*. Trans. Robert Hurley, Mark Seem and Helen Lane (Minneapolis: University of Minnesota Press, 1983), p. 270.
18. Danuza Machado, Phobia and Perversion. *Journal of the Centre for Freudian Analysis and Research* 2, 1993.

19. These are only a few of the stories Anjali shared about animals. She also spoke of parrots and cats in equally idiosyncratic and often sensuous terms. The clinician often found herself unmoored by the strangeness of these stories, a sentiment echoed by her Lacanian supervisor. Anjali spoke about staying up late 'washing the hamster' and 'petting the parrot,' neither of which she found to be odd behaviors for the animals noted in the least. In fact, she seemed completely perplexed by the punctuation of these phrases and inquiry into these moments explicitly describing contact with the nonhuman.
20. While the clinician had considered Anjali's previous statement that her mother was always 'spying' on her in her room and wondered as to its possible connections with 'bugs in [her] room' and the spider dream, Anjali herself did not have any associations herself to spiders in particular or 'spying' at this point, and so the clinician did not go further and make this connection or interpretation.
21. Cf. Jennifer Matthews, The Clinical Structure of Phobia: Lacan's Reformulation of the Variables of Its Treatment (unpublished master's thesis, Middlesex University. London, 2010).
22. Hans. Angelaki: *Journal of the Theoretical Humanities* 2(12): 69–79, 2007.
23. Ibid., p. 76.
24. Gilles Deleuze and Felix Guattari, *A Thousand Plateaus: Capitalism and Schizophrenia*, trans. Brian Massumi (London: Continuum, 1987), p. 256.

Bibliography

Deleuze, Gilles, and Felix Guattari. 1983. *Anti-Oedipus: Capitalism and Schizophrenia*. Trans. Robert Hurley, Mark Seem, and Helen Lane. Minneapolis: University of Minnesota Press.

———. 1987. *A Thousand Plateaus: Capitalism and Schizophrenia*. Trans. B. Massumi. London: Continuum.

Fink, Bruce. 1997. *A Clinical Introduction to Lacanian Psychoanalysis: Theory and Technique*. Cambridge: Harvard University Press.

Freud, Sigmund. 1953. Analysis of a Phobia in a Five-Year-Old Boy. In *Sigmund Freud: Collected Papers, Vol. 3*, ed. Ernest Jones. Trans. A. Stratchey and J. Strachey. New York: Basic Books.

Hook, Derek, and Calum Neill. 2008. Perspectives on 'Lacanian Subjectivities'. *Subjectivity* 24 (1): 247–255.

Lacan, Jacques. 1957. *The Seminar of Jacques Lacan, Book IV: The Object Relation*. Trans. L.V.A. Roche, unpublished manuscript, ed. Jacques-Alain Miller.

Machado, Danuza. 1993. Phobia and Perversion. *Journal of the Centre for Freudian Analysis and Research* 2.

Matthews, Jennifer. 2010. *The Clinical Structure of Phobia: Lacan's Reformulation of the Variables of Its Treatment.* Unpublished master's thesis, Middlesex University, London.

Palomera, Vincente. 1992. The Paternal Function and Little Hans' Phobia. *Newsletter of the Freudian Field* 6 (1–2): 49–61.

Pluth, Ed. 2007. On Sexual Difference and Sexuality 'as such': Lacan and the Case of Little Hans. *Angelaki: Journal of the Theoretical Humanities* 2 (12): 69–79.

The Human Not in the Human

A. Kiarina Kordela

The Subject–Object of Commodity Fetishism

If today we speak of the posthuman condition or the subject qua subject–object, and if bodies of knowledge and science make it possible to enable the existence of humans as living organisms with intraspecies biological and machinic components, it is because in the capitalist mode of production humans become inseparable from the means and the products of production,[1] which by now range from plants and animals to machines and biogenetically produced life, to information, language, and affects. When Jacques Lacan says that 'man thinks with his object,' we must take him literally—*man thinks with his product.*[2] Karl Marx spells out more clearly Lacan's point in his notorious theory of commodity fetishism.

This chapter was originally published as 'The Subject-Object of Commodity Fetishism, Biopolitics, Immortality, Sacrifice, and Bioracism' in a special issue of *Cultural Critique*, vol. 96 (Spring 2017): 37–70. We thank the editors for giving us permission to reprint the essay.

A.K. Kordela (✉)
Macalester College, Saint Paul, MN, USA

G. Basu Thakur, J.M. Dickstein (eds.), *Lacan and the Nonhuman*,
The Palgrave Lacan Series, DOI 10.1007/978-3-319-63817-1_4

The radically new and, as Marx calls it, 'mysterious' 'character of the product of labour—as soon as it assumes the form of a commodity'—lies in 'the fact that the commodity reflects the social characteristics of men's own labour as *objective characteristics of the products* of labour themselves, as the *socio-natural properties of these things*.'[3] While struggling to grasp this mysterious phenomenon in *Capital, Volume 1*, Marx can barely believe his own words when he writes that 'the fetishism of the commodity' designates the fact that a 'definite social relation between men themselves…assumes here, for them, the fantastic form of a relation between things,' or that 'to the producers…the social relations between their private labours appear…as material [*dinglich*—thingly] relations between persons and social relations between things.'[4]

As Étienne Balibar comments in his *La Philosophie de Marx* (1993), this fetishistic inversion is paradoxically possible not because of the thingliness or materiality of the commodities, but because 'commodities,' while being 'useful material objects…also possess another quality, which is immaterial but no less objective: their exchange-'alue…expressed…as a certain sum of money,' which, as Georg Simmel stressed, is 'a mere symbol, neutral as regards its intrinsic value'; it is 'an idea which is embodied in a representative symbol.'[5] What astonishes Marx is his discovery that, through their value, 'the products of labour become commodities'; that is, in Marx's words, '*socio-natural* properties'—'*sensuous* things which are at the same time *supra-sensible* or *social*,' use-values, or material things—are at the same time exchange-values, immaterial symbols, or signs. Therefore, as Marx concludes, the relations of the commodities themselves constitute people's own 'language'—that is, people's thoughts.[6] The vicissitudes of the relations of the commodities are reflected as the vicissitudes of the relations of the signs to which the speaking subject is subjected. The mind thinks like capital thinks.

As a result, as Balibar writes, the fact that 'value…confer[s] on [the commodity] an added objectivity' means that it is 'the "objective laws" of the circulation of commodities' that 'determine[s] the conditions [of the] individuals,' whereby 'the *personalities* of the individuals' become '*quite irrelevant*.'[7] Therefore, Balibar continues, what makes Marx's 'theory of fetishism…one of the greatest theoretical constructions of modern philosophy' is that it shows 'that there is no theory of objectivity without a theory of subjectivity. *By rethinking the constitution of social objectivity,*

Marx at the same time virtually revolutionized the concept of the "subject."'[8] Commodity fetishism means, Balibar says, that 'the constitution of the world is not...the work of a subject, but a genesis of subjectivity (*a* form of determinate historical subjectivity) as part (and counterpart) of the social world of objectivity.'[9]

This is why in his reading of Hegel, Alexandre Kojève states that the laborer 'contemplates himself when he contemplates [his product].'[10] In other words, commodity fetishism means that, once in capitalism, we are in a domain in which, again in Balibar's words, *the relations of the objects* 'constitute subjects or forms of subjectivity and consciousness *in* the very field of objectivity.' In short, commodity fetishism means that in a commodified world there are no humans as opposed to products, but human-products or product-humans—subject–objects. The advent of the capitalist mode of production already heralds the death of the transcendent subject, while it provides the conditions that sooner or later necessitated its invention.

For, although commodity fetishism and its corollary, the subject–object, are intrinsic to the essence of capitalism as such—that is, of capitalism as a set of potentialities that are not all actualized at their fullest from the outset but, rather, actualize themselves to various degrees at diverse historical moments. It is only after a certain development of capitalism that their actualization attained the critical mass required for them to become self-conscious. Also, it is because of the lack of such self-consciousness prior to this moment that both the subject and power were conceived as transcendent. Balibar makes the difference between these two stages of capitalism clear by distinguishing two phases in Marx's work.[11]

Marx's early phase of *The German Ideology* corresponds to the former period of capitalism, in which power is perceived as predicated on the function of ideology, while his later phase, marked by *Capital*, represents the latter period of capitalism as a system of full-fledged commodity fetishism. In both cases, fetishism and ideology, Balibar explains, there occurs a 'splitting up of the real community of individuals,' that

> ...is followed by a projection or transposition of the social relation onto an external 'thing,' a third term. Only, in the one case [ideology], the thing is an 'idol,' an abstract representation which seems to exist all on its own in the ethereal realm of ideas (Freedom, Justice, Humanity, Law), whereas in

> the other [fetishism] it is a 'fetish,' a material thing which seems to belong to the earth, to nature, while exerting an irresistible power over individuals (the commodity and, above all, money).[12]

Ideology is marked by a dualism between immanence and transcendence, the earthly world and the 'ethereal realm of ideas,' which is why 'the theory of ideology is fundamentally a *theory of the State* (by which we mean the mode of domination inherent in the State),' and, accordingly, its corollary view regarding 'the conditions and objectives of the revolutionary struggle' is that 'of overthrowing a bourgeois domination which has entered into contradiction with the development of civil society.'[13]

Here domination is perceived as emanating from a realm above or transcendent to civil society. By contrast, in the world of the fetish, it is the earthly material thing that assumes a supernatural and, thus, 'irresistible power over individuals.' Commodity fetishism folds transcendence completely within the plane of immanence, which is both why it marks the full actualization of secularization and why 'fetishism is fundamentally a *theory of the market* (the mode of subjection or constitution of the "world" of subjects and objects inherent in the organization of society as market and its domination by market forces).'[14]

With the shift from ideology (State) to fetishism (market), we pass from the question of domination to the problematic of 'subjection,' not simply in the sense of subjugation but, foremost, in the sense of subjectivation or the 'constitution' of both subjects and—beause the subject is the counterpart of the object—objects, as precisely subject–objects. This is what Balibar means when he writes that 'Marx's *The German Ideology* is a theory of the constitution of *power*, whereas what is described in *Capital*, by way of its definition of fetishism, is a mechanism of subjection.'[15]

Moreover, this 'mechanism of subjection' corresponds to the power that Foucault refers to when he speaks of a 'form of power [that] applies itself to immediate everyday life…a form of power' that does not simply 'subject [subjects] to someone else by control and dependence,' as was the case in State domination, but 'makes individuals subjects' and enables them to form their 'own identity by a conscience or self-knowledge.'[16] This power of everyday life is not transcendent but immanent, and it is the form of power Foucault would eventually call 'biopower'—the power proper to the self-conscious subject–object.

My reference to self-consciousness invites a clarification of a major Spinozian epistemological distinction that informs the methodology of the present work and that was hinted at in an earlier footnote. To put it crudely, implied in the argument here is the thesis that State and ideology are already forms of commodity fetishism, without knowing it, as it were. This is true, insofar as by this is *not* meant that the subjects under the power of the State and ideology are subjects with, what often has been called, a 'false consciousness'—that is, subjects incapable of understanding their real state of affairs; the real dynamics of power; and, further, the ways in which they are exploited, and so on.

The alternative to, or opposite of, self-consciousness is not false consciousness, for, to use Spinoza's own words, 'truth is the standard both of itself and of the false,' which is to say, truth lies also in the so-called false.[17] This is why Spinoza replaced the distinction between true and false consciousness with that between the virtual and the actual. The 'virtual' stands for the essence of the object in question, in this case capitalism.[18] Essentially, or on the level of the virtual, capitalism and commodity fetishism are inseparable, or, as Marx put it, 'fetishism…attaches itself to the products of labour, so soon as they are produced as commodities, and…is therefore inseparable from the production of commodities.'[19] Commodity fetishism emerges the moment a good is produced as a commodity; that is, as something for which exchange procures surplus-value, which is the case only within the capitalist mode of production.

Nevertheless, historically certain developments (e.g., massification, systematization, technologization, and so on) of the production of commodities are presupposed for commodity fetishism to take sufficient hold of a society; that is, for it to become conscious of the fact that it lives in the mode of commodity fetishism so that it becomes conscious of its essence, which is what I mean by saying that it becomes self-conscious. At this point, the potential of the mode of production in question, which has so far been known only on the virtual level, is sufficiently actualized to begin to become known gradually by the subjects who embody this mode of production. In other words, up to that moment subjects were not prey to some false consciousness; they were de facto incapable of knowing what was lurking all along on the virtual and was still manifesting itself only scarcely on the actual level, therefore, can be known only retroactively.

It follows that, although the full actualization of commodity fetishism historically postdates the emergence of secular capitalist modernity, taken as potentiality its inception already inaugurates the era in which a whole battery of discourses would be mobilized to construct the intrinsically modern notion of 'subjectivity'—that is, what transcends objectivity, at the very same time that 'subjectivity' would already have 'shifted'; as Balibar puts it, from 'its "transcendent"...position...into a position of effect or result of the social process.'[20] This is why in *Capital*—whose object of analysis is capitalism as an economic system in general, of which mercantilism, industrialism, and whatever stage of capitalism would come after it are only various degrees of actualization of the same system; Marx's sole mention of an autonomous or 'dominant subject [*übergreifendes Subjekt*]' refers to capital itself.[21]

Under this sole dominant subject, all other so-called subjects are counterparts of objects insofar as both are commodities—that is, again in Balibar's words, 'both a representation [exchange-value] and, at the same time, an object [use-value].'[22] Therefore, with capitalism, we are—essentially from the outset, and self-consciously at least since the mid-nineteenth century (Marx's *Capital, Volume 1,* was published in 1867) (i.e., since the earliest beginnings of modernism)—already after the subject. We are in the era of *the subject of commodity fetishism*; that is, *the subject–object* or *the subject-product*, which has *a double ontological status,* as *both a material use-value and an immaterial symbol or exchange-value.*

This double ontological status of the subject–object also entails a double temporality: qua use-value, the subject–object pertains to the finite linear or diachronic time in which everything is perishable or mortal; qua exchange-value or abstract symbol, by contrast, it is immortal and immune to physical decay. This double ontological status of the subject–object is the very precondition for the transformation of money into capital; that is, the accumulation of surplus-value—which again indicates that commodity fetishism constitutes an integral part of the essence of capital. In addition, as we have seen, the form of power that regulates the subject–object is biopower. This means that, just as the transcendent subject marks the consciousness of the subject prior to its self-consciousness as subject–object, the power of the State and ideology is the form of power prior to its self-consciousness as biopower.[23]

Human Biopolitics, or, the Politics of the One-Dimensional Biological Body

Even though this next section approaches biopower as a form of power that addresses subject–objects, its title refers to conceptualizations of biopower and biopolitics that have so far dominated the current discourse, and which, as will gradually become clear, do not take into account the double ontological status and temporality of the subject–object. What is here offers a brief recapitulation of such eminent theories of biopolitics.

Although Aristotle used the term *bios* to designate the specifically human aspect of life as a social and political animal, as opposed to *zoe* (life in its physical or biological sense that characterizes all animals), the term 'bios' reenters the contemporary theoretical discourse, through the neologisms *biopower* and *biopolitics*, to designate the *political* control of life in its *biological* sense. During the 1970s, Michel Foucault linked bios to political power to indicate a transformation in power's mechanisms beginning in the seventeenth century, in which political control over 'juridical' matters extended to include and focus primarily on the 'biological existence of a population.' The old sovereignty, as 'the right of seizure of things, time, bodies, and ultimately life itself,' gradually yielded to 'the administration of bodies and the calculated management of life,' with its various 'disciplines of the body' and 'the regulations of the population' as to its 'propagation, births…mortality…health, life expectancy and longevity'—all of which are functions aimed at enhancing the life of a physical or biological body.[24]

The Italian philosopher Giorgio Agamben stresses further the notion of 'bios' as the physical fact of life by returning to Aristotle and invoking the other Greek term, '*zoe*,' which indicates the undifferentiated, presymbolic, or 'bare life' as opposed to *bios* in the Aristotelian sense of organized political life. For Agamben, Foucault's hegemonic 'liberal-democratic State' is destined since the politicization of 'birth' (i.e., of 'bare natural life as such')—evidenced in the first of the 1789 Declarations: 'Men are born and remain free and equal in rights'—to become, through the logic of 'blood and soil,' totalitarian.[25] For, Agamben continues, the Jews 'were exterminated not in a mad and giant [sacrificial] holocaust but, exactly as Hitler had announced, "as lice," which is to say, as bare life,' so that the 'dimension in which the extermination took place is neither religion nor law, but biopolitics'—a dimension in which life is bare, severed from the Symbolic function of the Signifier, and thus the Law.[26]

Drawing on Hannah Arendt, Agamben argues that 'Foucault never brought his insights to bear on…the exemplary place of modern biopolitics: the politics of the great totalitarian states of the twentieth century' and 'the concentration camp,' the victims of which were not unlike the *hominess sacri* (a concept introduced by Roman Law), insofar as both the victim of the Holocaust and the *homo sacer* are marked by '*the unpunishability of [their] killing and the ban on [their] sacrifice.*'[27] In the twentieth century, Agamben concludes, 'the concentration camp' becomes 'the new biopolitical nomos [law] of the planet.'[28]

What the following argues is that, far from the physical and material fact of the body, *bios* and *biopolitics concern the subject–object's relation to the specific modes of temporality introduced by the advent of capitalism*, which include but are not limited to those pertaining to the double ontological status of the subject–object, and which surreptitiously reintroduce fantasies of immortality. So, we must first identify the modes of temporality that emerge in the secular capitalist era. For this reason, the next section returns to Marx, and specifically to his theory of labor-power, and the subsequent section links Marx to Aristotle to describe the fourth and last temporality that marks secular capitalist modernity.

Bios, or, Labor-Power, or, the Power of Self-Actualization

The generalized 'fixed' idea, Marx writes, that, with capitalism, economy is no longer dependent on slavery but on 'free' laborers introduced an unforeseen transformation in the nature of labor. Marx elaborates on this fact in *Capital, Volume 1*, but already in the *Grundrisse* he had noted that the difference between slavery or serfdom—as practiced throughout the antiquity and feudalism—and free labor—as practiced in capitalism—is that the latter case involves buying and selling labor-power. Capitalism is based on the central commodity of labor-power, which, Marx writes, is 'the use-value which the worker has to offer to the capitalist…[and which] is *not materialized* in a product, does not exist apart from him at all, thus exists *not really*, but only *in potentiality*.'[29]

Since the inception of capitalism with its 'free' workers, labor-power is 'potentiality'; that is, nothing actual but the *sheer power* of labor *to actualize* itself in a product. *Potentiality or the power of self-actualization* goes to the market and gets commodified. As Paolo Virno remarks, labor-power designates the '*ability* to work,' and as such, 'labor-power incarnates (literally) a fundamental category of philosophical thought: specifically, the potential'—that is, 'that which is *not present*' but a '*possibility* [that] is bought and sold' so that potentiality 'becomes…an exceptionally important commodity.'[30] Labor-power, therefore, Virno continues, 'is not separable from the *living person* of the…worker' who 'is the substratum of that labor-power which, in itself, has no existence.'[31] The body and life understood as 'pure and simple *bios*, acquires a specific importance [in capitalism] in as much as it is the tabernacle…of mere potential.'[32] It is *as potentiality or the power of self-actualization that* bios *becomes the object of biopolitics in capitalist modernity*.

It follows that, *pace* Michel Foucault, the primary task of biopolitics is not to control the '*biological* existence of a population' and 'the random element inherent in biological processes' (e.g., 'procreation,' 'heredity,' etc.).[33] Nor is it Giorgio Agamben's 'bare natural life.'[34] Rather, *the target of biopolitics is the body as the bearer of labor-power—bios qua power of self-actualization*.

It is no accident that the first modern philosopher—as is acknowledged even by the one who would eventually become his philosophical adversary, Hegel—Spinoza introduced the power of self-actualization as nothing less than the One substance, which is 'God or Nature [*deus sive natura*].'[35] Spinoza's conception of God is properly secular insofar as it replaces the creationist assumption of a supernatural God with *a nature capable of actualizing itself*—that is, with nature qua potentiality. Through Spinoza we understand that the *capitalist commodification of labor-power amounts to the capitalist commodification of God*, which constitutes *the basis of what we call 'secularization.'*

The concomitant of this commodification is *the secularization* of a further temporality appropriated by capitalism: *divine temporality* (i.e., eternity). For, qua bios or labor-power, our bodies live in 'eternity' because, being the power of its self-actualization, bios, like Spinoza's substance, is of an 'eternal nature' that is 'necessary and not…contingent' and, thus, exists 'under a species of eternity [*sub specie aeternitatis*].'[36] The power of self-actualization that we call bios enters the historical realm of secular capitalist modernity under the species of eternity—and thereby secularizes eternity as a metaphysical category that can be bought and sold on the market.

It is crucial, for reasons to which this chapter returns later, not to conflate eternity with infinite or indefinite duration. For duration pertains to actualized existence (what Spinoza calls modes of substance), whereas eternity pertains to potentiality (i.e., Spinoza's attributes of substance). As Gilles Deleuze writes, duration 'is the continuation of existence from a beginning onward.'[37] 'It involves a beginning' and, although it does not involve a *necessary* 'end,' the 'end of a duration, which is to say, death.' Nevertheless, this comes 'from the encounter of the existing mode with another mode that decomposes' it—which is what makes living beings mortal.[38]

In other words, 'duration contrasts with eternity because eternity' pertains only to 'a full…*power* of acting,' whereas duration pertains to what is already actualized by the full power of acting.[39] This, in turn, is to say that bios pertains to eternity but does *not* mean that we live in infinite duration, which would amount to *being immortal*; however, our mind, like capital, 'understands [the Body] not [only] from the fact that it conceives the Body's present actual existence, but [also] from the fact that it conceives the Body's essence under a species of eternity'—that is, as the power of acting or labor-power.[40] Also in capitalism, as we have seen, this power is bought and sold on the market.

Secular Immortality, or, the Surplus-Enjoyment of Subject–Objects

Prior to capitalism, the total amount of available money could increase only by producing additional coinage, but not by the mere act of exchange, which is why those modes of production constituted economic systems of equilibrium. As in the principle of the conservation of energy in physics, the amount of money initially advanced and the amount of money eventually collected in any given set of economic transactions remained the same—it was simply the unequal distribution of a fixed amount of money, predicated on lineages of ancestry, that made some people richer than others. The fact that capitalism procures, and is defined by precisely the fact that its transactions result in accumulating, surplus-value means that it is a system of disequilibrium—here we are in the realm of entropy. Consequently, beyond secularizing and commodifying eternity, secular capitalist modernity and its systemic disequilibrium established a hitherto aberrant mode of temporality as the norm, which is the specific temporality of surplus-value to which we shall presently turn. As we shall also see, the introduction of this unforeseen temporality transmogrified feasible enjoyment into surplus-enjoyment—that is, an enjoyment that, like capital, is never satisfied in itself and always strives for more of itself.

Many may recognize 'surplus-enjoyment' as a term introduced by Lacan, but its logic and temporality were already described by Aristotle in his examination of what we could call the proto-form of capitalism—namely, the then limited and widely condemned practice of *chrematistics* (i.e., the trade or money-lending for the purpose of making more money), as opposed to *oikonomia* (i.e., the acquisition of just the goods required for household-management).[41] Just as Lacan fashioned surplus-enjoyment against the blueprint of surplus-value—properly following the logic of commodity fetishism, according to which, if capitalism's unique characteristic is the accumulation of surplus-value, then the unique characteristic of human subjectivity within capitalist modernity also must involve a surplus. Aristotle, too, grasped the logic of surplus-enjoyment by intuiting the logic of surplus-value, as it could be glimpsed through the practice of chrematistics in antiquity.

Prior to turning to Aristotle's account of surplus-enjoyment, however, let us examine the peculiar temporality of surplus-value. It is the fourth mode of temporality involved in the workings of the capitalist mode of production, next to: (1) eternity, as the temporality of bios qua potentiality; (2) the temporality of use-value (the material object) and of actual bodies; and (3) the temporality of exchange-value, as the sign that represents the material object. Use-value exists in the linear and finite time in which material objects and bodies undergo physical decay. As use-value, the commodity requires its specific labor (i.e., a unique, specialized activity) that is bound to specific materials and takes place within a finite span of time that lasts from the beginning of production to the moment the commodity enters circulation and becomes abstract exchange-value.

This time of the use-value is what Marx calls 'production time,' and corresponds to what in linguistics Ferdinand de Saussure calls 'diachrony,' the time in which language changes because of nonsystemic historico–cultural changes. The moment the commodity enters circulation, it becomes an exchange-value (i.e., something that can be exchanged for anything else), regardless of the object's specific inherent qualities that, as a matter of fact, no longer exist. For, as Marx stresses, 'not an atom of matter enters into the objectivity of commodities as values; in this [they are] the direct opposite of the coarsely sensuous objectivity of commodities as physical objects.'[42] Here we are in the realm of abstract and arbitrary—that is, as presently will be clarified, secular signs. These are signs, which as we know from Saussure, that establish themselves in differential relations with all other signs, in 'synchrony' (i.e., what Marx calls 'circulation time')—a mode of temporality that, unlike diachrony, does not involve any linear passage of time.

Saussure's conceptualization of the sign expressly parallels the constitution of exchange-value and is for this reason specifically secular. Having stated that the sign is determined not only by its signification but also by its 'linguistic value,' Saussure proceeds to explain by invoking precisely economic value:

> Let us observe from the outset that even outside language all values are apparently governed by the same paradoxical principle. They are always composed:
>
> 1. of a *dissimilar* thing that can be *exchanged* for the thing of which the value is to be determined; and
> 2. of *similar* things that can be *compared* with the thing of which the value is to be determined.
>
> Both factors are necessary for the existence of a value.

To determine what a five-franc piece is worth one must therefore know: (1) that it can be exchanged for a fixed quantity of a different thing (e.g., bread); and (2) that it can be compared with a similar value of the same system (e.g., a one-franc piece), or with coins of another system (e.g., a dollar, etc.). In the same way, a word can be exchanged for something dissimilar, an idea; besides, it can be compared with something of the same nature, another word. Its value is therefore not fixed so long as one simply states that…it has this or that signification; one must also compare it with similar values, with other words that stand in opposition to it. Its content is really fixed only by the concurrence of everything that exists outside it.[43]

It is for this reason that the sign is both differential and 'arbitrary in that it actually has no natural connection with the signified.'[44] The rapture of the natural, and thus necessary, connection between Signifier and signified is what renders the sign secular. Foucault illustrates the difference between the presecular 'Word' and the secular sign by calling the former 'ternary' and the latter 'binary.' Whereas the presecular 'ternary sign' is based on 'the similitudes' which, because of their divine origin and guarantee, 'link the marks to the things designated by them' in an 'organic' or natural way, the secular 'binary sign' arrives after 'the destruction of the organic,' which renders the link between marks and things arbitrary.[45]

Returning now to the modes of temporality involved in the capitalist mode of production, while production time is marked, as Marx writes, by '*continuity*,' circulation time 'is the *interruption* of continuity contained in the character of capital as circulating,' and the tendency of which is '*circulation without… time*'—that is, simultaneity or synchronicity, a mode of time in which the instant and infinity coincide.[46] Matter exists only in production time, which is the exclusive realm in which commodities, including commodified laborers, are subject to physical decay and mortality. By contrast, circulation time does not involve any passage of time at all, and it is rather a flat slice of space in which infinity springs out of the instant at the same moment that the instant sucks infinity back into it, without any passage of time. This constitutes the first way in which capitalism brings infinity into the earthly world of economic exchange, and thereby renders it secular.

Surplus-value, however, takes infinity one step further. The accumulation of surplus-value cannot occur either in the finite diachrony of production time or in the synchronic infinity of circulation. For, in actual experience, it takes *a passage of time* for the total sum of value available in each slice of synchronic circulation to increase. In addition, because the vocation of capital, in Marx's words, is to be 'money which is worth more money,' this passage of time must go on infinitely.[47] Therefore, surplus-value presupposes a sort of valve, as it were, that releases infinity out of its legitimate realm of circulation (i.e., the spatial disc) and lets it flow into diachrony—a realm that is, by definition, finite—so that *what takes place in continuous time can endure infinitely* and, as far as life is concerned, *immortally*. As opposed to the finite diachrony of production time, the infinite duration of surplus-value is the linear, yet perforated, time of the perpetual succession of synchronic discs of circulation required for surplus-value to accrue infinitely.

In this way, surplus-value, as Éric Alliez puts it, 'open[s] up the duration of the durable' to infinity, and thereby surplus-value defeats the primordial nature of the durable to remain, however long-lasting and resilient it may be, always confined within its finite durance and mortal.[48] Thus, surplus-value redoubles the secularization of infinity, this time as the limitless duration of the undead. *Surplus-value secularizes immortality*. In its ever-ascending or *descending* spiral—for economic crises are necessary too (debt is the inverted mirror image of surplus-value)—the time of infinite duration unfolds by leaps, perpetually taking us from one synchronic disc of circulation to the next, ad infinitum or *immortaliter*.

Parenthetically, because debt will eventually become a center of our attention later, the reason why I emphatically added the word '*descending*' in the preceding statement is that economic crises are not only necessary for the advancement of capitalism, as Marx already knew, but also that debt, as mentioned earlier, is the inverted mirror image of surplus-value, insofar as it, too, is a form of disequilibrium. For capitalist debt is not like the debt of precapitalist economic systems, which was determined not by the contingencies of the arbitrary fluctuations of a market (as in the capitalist sense) but by natural fecundity or dearth and the predestination of pedigree—and possibly other marginal contingencies, which, again, related not to systemic (market) itineraries but to what one could still legitimately call individual fates. The fact that capitalism enabled an unforeseen social mobility in terms of wealth means both that it introduced what was to become the American dream and an equally Cinderella-like leap to indebtedness.

For now, however, let us return to the fact that commodity fetishism necessitates that this capitalist introduction of infinite duration into the realm of the actual does not limit itself within economic surplus-value, because in the capitalist universe there is no dualism between economic objects and human subjects. It is this insight that Aristotle tacitly grasped when he recognized the effects of infinite duration on human enjoyment. Aristotle's analysis begins with a comparison between *oikonomia* or 'household-management' (i.e., the practice of exchange dominant at his time) to *chrematistics* (i.e., trade or money-lending to acquire profit or interest)—that is, an intimation of capitalism as still an aberrant or 'unnatural' practice.

The end or purpose of exchange in oikonomia is defined, Aristotle writes, 'by the proper use of the article in question,' which is always limited, such as the use of a 'shoe' which is to 'put [it] on your foot.'[49] By contrast, chrematistics or the 'form of money-making' is not part of nature because it is concerned with 'how the greatest profits might be made out of the exchanges,' and 'there is indeed no limit to the amount of riches to be got from this mode' of exchange.[50] Unlike oikonomia, which is natural, chrematistics, Aristotle concludes, is unnatural because 'there is no limit to the end which this kind of acquisition has in view.'[51] This is why, as Marx puts it, the 'circulation of money as capital is an end in itself,' and that the 'circulation of capital is...limitless.'[52]

Natural oikonomia is the sister of the natural or organic link between the Signifier and the signified, whereas unnatural chrematistics intimates the collapse of this link and its entire (presecular) onto-epistemology. If Aristotle abhors the limitless exchange that is, by definition, an end of itself, it is because he also grasps that its consequences extend beyond economy to inflict itself on his entire worldview. For, the establishment of limitless accumulation of profit as the dominant mode of exchange would entail the collapse of the basic Aristotelian onto-epistemological premise—*entelechy*—which, through its itinerary across countries on all sides of the Mediterranean, survived antiquity to become also the cornerstone of the variants of monotheism. 'Entelechy' is the idea that everything bears within itself its own *telos*. More specifically, entelechy postulates, in Aristotle's words, that 'the *means* towards the end are not unlimited' because 'the end itself [is] setting the limit in each case.' Everything has its specific limited 'telos,' of which it is the means, and the means cannot coincide with the end.[53]

The limitless movement of capital as self-valorizing value defies this principle of entelechy wholesale, for it is not just value that becomes its own end but also everything else becomes exchange-value, serving nothing other than this same unlimited end of value to valorize itself; thus, it is deprived of any possible entelechy as a distinct thing. As Marx put it, that 'the movement of capital is…limitless' is tantamount to the fact that 'the circulation of money as capital is an end in itself'; it 'is tautological' or 'a roundabout way of exchanging money for money, the same for the same, and appears to be an operation as purposeless as it is absurd.'[54] Once the end becomes the accumulation of surplus-value, the sole real *telos* of the shoe, as of any commodity, becomes to exchange it for the sake of accruing ever more value.

Aristotle's shoe, the purpose of which is to wear it on your foot, is presecular, and what he vociferously attacks is a practice, which was to become eventually what we today know as capitalism; through this the shoe loses its specific entelechy and becomes a value in a limitless movement, the aim of which is the perpetual accumulation of value. At that moment, the shoe becomes part of a nature that is secular—a nature that *is* a self-valorizing value, as much as it is the power of self-actualization. Once the perpetual accumulation of value emerges, a shoe can be neither worn nor can it wear out; it is as undead as the posthumanity to which it belongs. In this realm, to claim, as Aristotle did, that the shoe is something other than self-valorizing value, that it has some other *telos* of its own, would amount to a sacrilege of the whole condition of secular capitalist posthumanity—namely, its inviolable principle of being the power of self-actualization.

The power of self-actualization, however, is insatiable and greedy. For, although both oikonomia and chrematistics (i.e., capitalism) are 'concerned with the same thing, property'; in the latter case, 'the end is sheer increase' so that 'some people…imagine…and never cease to believe that their store of coined money ought to be…increased without limit. …*Desire for life being unlimited, they desire also an unlimited amount of what enables it to go on.*'[55] Thus, instead of engaging in the production of goods, they engage in the purchase and selling (i.e., the circulation) of goods, 'for *where enjoyment consists in excess, men look for that skill which produces the excess that is enjoyed.*'[56]

Once enjoyment becomes excess (i.e., surplus-enjoyment) one can derive it only in the infinite duration that perpetually propels individuals from one synchronic disc of circulation to another, and thereby satisfies a yearning for unlimited circulation and life. By engaging in circulation, we partake in the illusion of immortality—an illusion that, with the dominance of chrematistics in the form of capitalism, was destined to become the modern secular mode of immortality. The bait of biopower remains profoundly presecular (i.e., immortality), but it promises it in a secular fashion, as the immortality of the actual flesh that lives in diachrony.

To have access to immortality, however, one must exist neither as a physical body in the realm of production and its finite duration nor as labor-power in the virtual realm of potentiality and its eternity, but in the realm of the ever-proliferating discs of the circulation of exchange-values in whose infinite duration surplus-value accrues. In other words, one must constantly engage in consumerism, buying and selling, and, what is more, one must do so by aiming *not at the satisfaction of any needs but at the immediate renewal, the ideally ceaseless sustenance of consumerism itself.*

Now, we can comprehend more fully the workings of biopolitics, as the form of power that takes hold of the subjects of commodity fetishism. These are subjects whose bodies qua potentiality exist *sub specie aeternitatis*, yet, as actual physical bodies in duration, are mortal. Nonetheless, when in the realm of circulation, they become immortal. Insofar as its aim is the sustenance of the status quo (capitalism), biopolitics' true object, therefore, concerns the relation between the body as eternity (labor-power) and the body as (imagined) immortal actuality (i.e., the body that derives surplus-enjoyment). At the same instant that eternity is secularized in the form of labor-power, its *commodification deprives the subject-object of its own eternity and offers as its surrogate* the temporality of the effects of commodification (i.e., surplus-value and surplus-enjoyment) that is *infinite diachrony*, which constitutes the form of *immortality proper to the posthuman subject–object* of secular capitalist modernity.

In the act of consuming, subjects are not after either the satisfaction of needs or the fulfillment of desires, nor do they pursue pragmatist purposes, such as the acquisition of profit or anything else that could benefit their actual existence, except the latter's unconditional perpetuation. Their motivation is metaphysical, and the whole reduction of capitalism to utilitarianism, pragmatism, and cynicism is thoroughly misleading. For the life of the subject–object of biopower—*bios—is itself fundamentally metaphysical because its true temporality is eternity*. Thus, it lends itself more easily to the blinding fascination of the illusion of immortality than to the pursuit of any practical good. A fortiori, biopower exploits the fact that the subjects of commodity fetishism are willing to sacrifice everything to the altar of their source of immortality—circulation. This becomes particularly evident at moments of crisis and debt, when the act of consumerism cannot possibly yield any practical profit to the individual.

Sacrifice

Like surplus-value, debt increases its own power, or realizes its own vocation, not by finding an ultimate enjoyment (reaching a limit) but by incessantly accumulating. Just as there is accumulation of capital, there is accumulation of debt. For this reason, I conclude this line of argument by turning to Richard Dienst's *The Bonds of Debt: Borrowing Against the Common Good*, which, motivated by Deleuze's statement that in control societies 'a man is no longer a man confined but a man in debt,' raises indebtedness to a defining characteristic of not only economic crisis, sovereign or individual, but also of the human condition.[57] Dienst argues that capitalism distributes debt in exploitative ways and, as a solution, he proposes 'Jubilee' (i.e., 'the total cancelation of debts'), an idea first 'articulated' within the 'Judeo-Christian world…in the twenty-fifth book of Leviticus.'[58]

Dienst also links this call for cancelation of debts to Walter Benjamin's 'Theses on the Philosophy of History,' summarizing them as follows:

> Whereas the history of the oppressors conveys the continuity of obligations, embodied in material things and historical concepts, the tradition of the oppressed teaches the strategy of interruption and disconnection, the moment of flashing up and breaking apart. In such a moment, all bets are off and all debts are cancelled.[59]

Dienst is fully aware that 'such events can never simply start over at zero,' that 'there is something positively schizo about the *Jetztzeit*,' and that, of course, 'Benjamin knows this complexity inside out,' for as the next passage cited from Benjamin on the same page clearly indicates: 'We claim from those born later not thanks for our victories but rather remembrance for our defeats.'[60]

Still, whether we expect 'thanks for victories' or 'remembrance for defeats,' in either case we render the future indebted to us, just as whether it is profit or debt that accumulates, both are different expressions of surplus—that is, of a system based on disequilibrium, whether negative or positive. Besides, like Benjamin, Dienst, after all, is not really arguing for a total elimination of debt; rather he is arguing for a nonexploitative redistribution of debt among ourselves. But such an egalitarian distribution can be realized only in a world populated by enlightened subjects who acknowledge others as their equals. What the following examines is whether the solution proposed through this reference to Jubilee (inadvertently) falls into a trap set up by the discourse of enlightened secular modernity itself because, as the stage of capitalist actualization enables one to recognize, at stake is not the transcendent human subject, as constructed by the discourse of Enlightenment, but the posthuman subject–object of commodity fetishism and of biopolitics.

I concur with Dienst that the fact that during times of economic crisis there is a '*proliferation of shopping spaces*[, which] should be seen as the physical extension of the regime of indebtedness, where individual subjects are empowered to enact their own *fidelity to the reigning powers of money*,' by offering to it not only the last penny they have but also pence they do not have.[61] This occurs, as Dienst argues, in the collective sacrificial ritual of shopping and of indebting oneself to credit cards; yet, I would add, this is not just in order to enact one's fidelity to the divinity of money but also in order to have access to immortality. This immortality is not a private affair but rather presupposes the collective flow of the market.

As Dienst writes:

> [S]hopping embraces the basic contradiction of consumerism, offering a way to bear being in debt, turning endless obligations into fleeting enjoyment, staking a claim in a collective excess that would be inaccessible to mere individuals.[62]

Shopping provides access to the temporality of the infinite duration of synchronic circulations—something that requires not individuals but an endless concatenation of members in the collective flow of circulation. Which is why, for all the talk about individualism in capitalist modernity, biopolitics constitutes not individuals but containers that are both the receptacles and dispensers of this flow.

Nevertheless, here too, as in the case of the shift from State/ideology to market/commodity fetishism, one must consider the various historical stages of actualization. Dienst helps one do so by revisiting a section from Deleuze and Guattari's *Anti-Oedipus* (1972), where, in his summary, he writes:

> [W]e find a sustained treatment of the historical forms of debt, organized in three major configurations. In the first, the so-called 'savage' system, debt is incurred and discharged through blood revenge and cruelty; in the 'despotic/barbarian' system, all debts are exercised as dispensations of the infinite credit of the divine ruler (it is the latter phases of this system that Foucault…call[s] 'sovereign society'); and finally, in the third system, which is capitalism as such, debts finally break free from the authority of the state and circulate across the whole social surface. Inheritance of the past ceases to be collective stockpiling or direct bequest, and instead takes shape as a private accumulation of capital.[63]

In the last configuration, debts and capital 'circulate across the whole social surface' and 'reciprocal responsibilities cease to be tied to lateral alliances or hierarchical obligations, and instead become subject to oscillating and optional transactions' so that 'henceforth there will be countless ways to be in debt, in all directions and according to various codes and protocols.'[64]

At stake, therefore, cannot be what Dienst's preceding passage calls 'a private accumulation of capital,' unless 'private' is understood in the structuralist sense of empty 'sites' that 'prevail over whatever occupies them.'[65] From a biopolitical perspective, the so-called 'private individual' is the void subject–object container through which certain amounts of capital or debt flow, depending on its position in relation to the rest of the sites constituting the whole social surface.[66] This is why when, in the next paragraph, Dienst recapitulates the three historical systems in terms of the 'social "eye"' or 'collective inscription of memory that keeps track of filiations and alliances, imposes duties, and records payments' in each, we note: 'In the first system, the memory is inscribed directly on the body, as a mark of pain; in the second, it is decreed by the Law; in the third, it circulates in the flows of money.'[67]

Extant theories of ideology and biopolitics, for which the body is considered as a biological entity linked to various degrees to the Law, address only the first two historical systems, even if they claim that biopolitics is specific to the third system of capitalist modernity. There is an affinity between the first two systems (i.e., the archaic and the sovereign) because of their being predicated on relatively similar, albeit also distinct, conceptions of the relation between transcendence and immanence, which contrasts them to the third system. To clarify this point, this section now turns to George Bataille's *Theory of Religion*, which offers a poignant account of the relationship between immanence and transcendence throughout history.

The archaic conception of the world as inhabited by spirits is based on an uninterrupted continuity of immanence and transcendence, on their effective overlap, even as some conceptual differentiation is already introduced. This is exemplified, Bataille argues, in the archaic 'positing of the things as subjects,' which entails that the 'virtues of a *thing*' consist in that it is '"capable of acting, thinking, and speaking" (just as men do).'[68] Consequently, even the 'positing…of a "supreme [transcendent] being"' can occur only as a positing '*in* the world.'[69]

Nevertheless, 'there is doubtless, in the invention of a supreme being, a determination to define a value that is greater than any other' so that 'there is no ultimate equality between' that being and any other being; for, 'by definition, the supreme being has the highest rank'. Still, 'all [beings] are of the same kind, in which immanence and personality are mingled; all can be *divine* and endowed with an operative power; all can speak the language of man. Thus, in spite of everything, they basically line up on a plane of equality.'[70] This is why in archaic societies, 'the world is still, in a fundamental way, immanence without a clear limit (an indistinct flow of being into being),' like 'water in water,' not unlike 'every animal [which too] *is in the world like water in water,*' knowing nothing of the transcendence of the subject to the object (e.g., in the 'way that we distinguish an object from ourselves'), acknowledging 'no transcendence between the eater and the eaten,' or anything that could 'introduce the relation of the master to the one he commands,' that 'might establish autonomy on one side and dependence on the other.'[71]

This world is presecular insofar as it involves a supreme supernatural being, yet, because all beings basically line up on 'a plane of equality,' beings pay their debts to themselves. That is, it is the being in its poor and paltry aspect as a 'profane tool' that pays its debt to itself in its aspect as a 'sacred' spirit.[72] This is why being in archaic societies necessitates an internal split between 'the reality of a profane world, of a world of things and bodies' and 'a holy and mythical world' of spirits.[73] Consequently, although 'within the limits of continuity, everything is spiritual' and 'there is no opposition of the mind and the body,' the mortal body, 'insofar as it is not present in sovereign spirits,' 'is gradually assimilated to the mass of things' so that 'real animals and plants separated from their spiritual truth slowly rejoin the empty objectivity of tools.'[74] Thus, 'animals, plants, tools, and other controllable things form a real world with the bodies that control them,' a world that, to be sure, remains 'subject to and traversed by divine forces,' yet is already 'fallen' so that only 'insofar as it is spirit, the human reality is holy, but it is profane insofar as it is real.'[75]

This is why the archaic being can pay its debt only to itself qua spirit and can do so only in the form of bloody sacrifice. For 'the thing—only the thing—is what sacrifice means to destroy in the victim,' as 'it draws the victim out of the world of utility and restores it to that of unintelligible caprice.'[76] If the distinction between profane tool and sacred spirit threatened to introduce a split in the continuity of being, sacrifice offers the antidote as a 'return to *intimacy*,' to the 'immanence between man and the world, between the subject and the object,' to the '*intimacy* of the divine world' of 'violent and uncalculated generosity'—the 'profound immanence of all that is.'[77]

It is in this sense that 'the first men were closer than we are to the animal world,' which is pure immanence, and the fact that 'nowadays Christians do not hesitate to recognize in the various "supreme beings" of which "primitives" have kept some memory, a first consciousness of the God they believe in'; this is the effect of oversimplifying reductionism.[78] For the shift from the mythical world of spirits to a divinity of a 'prestige comparable to that which the God of the Jews, and later that of the Christians, was to obtain' presupposes a process of fundamental sociopolitical and epistemological transformations, which we are not going to trace here.[79]

The point relevant to this chapter's topic is that in archaic societies biopolitics concerned directly the biological body—from the administration of sexuality as is evidenced in the laws concerning marriage, familial lines of inheritance, and so on, to the administration of death, as is evidenced in sacrifice—because the circulation of debts and their redemptions took place within the body, between its two aspects (i.e., the biological and the spiritual). 'Monotheism' and the politics of domination or sovereignty, on the other hand, inaugurated the paradigm in which biopolitics would continue to concern the biological body, but after the split between body and mind or spirit would have been established in terms of the opposition between immanence and absolute transcendence. By 'absolute' here is meant a transcendence according to which spirit is not only supernatural (which already was the case in archaic societies but only insofar as it also constituted the supernatural aspect of *nature* itself) but also is severed from nature, as its otherworldly or heavenly antipode.

This is the fundamental meaning of the split between body and mind. From then on, the Law will administer life and bodies to facilitate the redemption of debts to the transcendent divine infinite credit, which is why new, *blood-free,* forms of payment gradually began to prevail, forms that trained the biological body to withdraw into the background and let the mind ascend, however asymptotically, to spiritual transcendence. These forms include prayer, confession, meditation, and solitude (both as asceticism and incarceration), all of which would eventually lead to the secular modes of paying debts (e.g., meditation, self-reflection, and all the forms of regulation and administration). Foucault traces these from religious and policing mechanisms up to the establishment of modern philosophy, and the medicalization of the body and the mind (with its own, new, demands for asceticism). Yet, these modern secular variations of biopolitical redemption presuppose another major historical shift regarding the relationship between immanence and transcendence.

On the virtual level—that is, regardless of the historical development that may have been required for the full actualization of the potential of secular capitalist modernity—the shift from the presecular to the secular consists of a complete folding of transcendence within the plane of immanence so that even transcendent categories (e.g., eternity and so on) became immanent. This occurred through the replacement of spirit or divinity with *value*. Prior to secular capitalist modernity, the world had been conceived as consisting of two aspects, the material or natural and the immaterial or supernatural, whether the link between the two was cast in archaic/spiritual (i.e., continuity of immanence and transcendence) or sovereign/divine terms (i.e., dualism between immanence and transcendence). With the advent of capitalist value, the inherent division of the world into material and immaterial underwent a radical reconfiguration that untied it from the distinction between natural and supernatural.

Let us recall Marx's description of the material and the immaterial aspects of things, which, with capitalism, have become commodities: these are 'objects of utility' or 'use-values' (i.e., material things), while these 'sensuous things...are at the same time suprasensible or social' (i.e., 'values...as their [men's] language'[80]). However immaterial 'suprasensible' or social language and monetary symbols may be, they are not supernatural; with secularization, the counterpart of the natural became the cultural; and if up until modernism, the relationship between nature and culture was dualist or oppositional. In postmodernism it becomes monist, as the very concept of the posthuman subject–object indicates. The gradual secular obliteration of the natural–supernatural distinction took place as spirits, divinity, and their cognates yielded to value, both economic (exchange-value) and semantic (language or the Signifier).

This secular capitalist folding of transcendence into immanence may remind one more of archaic spiritualism rather than sovereign divinity because, both in spiritualism and in capitalism, the immaterial inheres in matter, and all material things are equal in this regard. Nonetheless, the difference remains; that is, the immaterial aspect of the thing is now disenchanted from its supernatural character—or, more accurately, it is *disenchanted consciously*. The similarity between the archaic and the secular capitalist paradigm is reflected in the fact that, in both, humans pay their debts to themselves. This is because, on the one hand, in archaic societies, as we have seen, beings sacrifice themselves in their aspect as profane tools to pay their debts to themselves in their aspect as 'sacred' spirits. On the other hand, in capitalism, to repeat Dienst's words, 'debts finally break free from the authority of the state' or any other transcendent agency, 'and circulate across the whole social surface' in the form of what appears to be 'private accumulation of capital.'[81]

Nevertheless, a major dissimilarity between the two systems remains, insofar as in secular capitalism everything that reeks of the supernatural eventually finds itself to be prevented from having access to consciousness—forever since Spinoza, Kant, and beyond, the primary postulate of secular enlightened reason has been precisely not to believe in superstition and anything supernatural. From this time, everything enchanted increasingly became the content of the unconscious, as Lacan's 'God is unconscious' was eventually to state explicitly.[82] Therefore, immortality—and, at least theoretically, all qualities attributed to divinity or spirits—can be fostered in the secular unconscious of the subject–object of commodity fetishism.

Even though on the virtual level this may be true of all capitalism, it is only with the shift from the State to the market that this is also historically fully actualized. At this point, the infinite credit of both the presecular spiritual or divine authorities and the (semi-secular) transcendent authority of the State/ideology is displaced onto the infinite credit of the capitalist market. Hereafter, as Dienst concludes, 'the market-eye keeps a watch over everything,' and it is this eye that—along with the eye of the 'media'—constitutes 'the organization of lived temporality around the interminable working-up and working-off of an imperishable indebtedness.'[83] Translated into the terms of the present chapter, Dienst's statement can be rewritten as: the market-eye constitutes the organization of lived temporality around the infinite diachrony of posthuman immortality.

Bioracism

This biopolitical organization of the lived temporality of the subject–object points to the possibility of a radical reconceptualization of racial discrimination. If shopping or consumption is the secular capitalist, and definitely the consciously posthuman bridge to the heavens of immortality, then, clearly, not everybody has equal access to it. As Dienst remarks on the basis of data given in the multi-authored *Harvard Design School Guide to Shopping*, 'the authors calculate that there is a global average of four square feet of retail space per person'; however, for instance, 'in the US, as always the world leader, there are thirty-one square feet per person.'[84]

If shopping enables the biopolitical constitution of subject–objects as those whose lived time assumes the form of the temporality of imperishable surplus or indebtedness, then a life that unfolds, mostly, let alone exclusively, in the finite diachrony of mortals would not count as human. *Immortality becomes the defining characteristic of the posthuman subject–object*, but not all 'humans' are posthumans; that is, not everybody has equal access to the gateway to immortality—shopping. As Foucault puts it, 'racism' is 'a break into the domain of life…between what must live and what must die.'[85] This break, which of course is defined in a different way in each historical system, also has undergone various stages of actualizations within its third, capitalist, modification.

In Foucault's words, 'from the seventeenth century onward' the break between what must live and what must die manifests itself as a 'racial war' and as a 'permanent struggle' that can assume several 'transcriptions'. For example, already in the seventeenth century, its 'first—*biological*—transcription'; or in 'the nineteenth century,' its 'second transcription' as 'class struggle'; and, finally, since the late nineteenth century as the 'way of establishing a biological-type caesura' of the 'evolutionist' (popularized Darwinian) type. This, for Foucault, seals the transcriptional itinerary of racism in secular capitalist modernity.[86]

This section concludes by suggesting that, once humanity is conscious of its posthumanity, we may find ourselves already in a fourth transcription of racism, one that we could call *socio-metaphysical and even socioreligious racism*. That is, religion being the past of what in modern Western philosophy was to become metaphysics, which is the full-fledged *bioracial* type of racism. In this actualized bioracial stage, the 'caesura' is defined *in terms of the relation of the subject–objects of society to its own metaphysical/religious categories*, specifically the infinite diachronic temporality of surplus or debt, as a surrogate for lost eternity—although relations to other metaphysical or religious categories also may lurk.

Even as Foucault's conception of bioracism did not go beyond evolutionism, he was the first to suggest that racism is 'the discourse of a battle that has to be waged not between races, but by *a* race that is portrayed as the one true race, the race that holds power and is entitled to define the norm, and against those who deviate from that norm…or pose a threat' to it.[87] In fact, Foucault continues, racism is 'a binary rift within society…the *splitting of a single race into a superrace and a subrace.…It is the reappearance, within a single race, of the past of that race*.'[88] More specifically, it is the splitting of a single race within the superrace of its consciousness and the subrace of its past that continues to be unconsciously active within the same race. In addition, the defense mechanism of a society against its own split entails the projection of its unconscious past onto the Other.

This is how today the dominant discourse of neoliberal capitalism ends up assuming not a secular but a secularist attitude; that is, both insentient to its unconscious perpetuation of its past and fanatically set against anything outside secular consciousness, which it recognizes only in its Other. It is no accident, then, that current movements of opposition to the status quo, peaceful and violent alike, tend toward a revival of spirituality or religiosity throughout the world. The unconscious is by definition unknowable for it is Real, but it is at least circumscribable. Plus, the only way for secularism to circumscribe its Real is to revisit its past.

Dienst is right to argue that 'the regime of indebtedness makes itself visible only in the parallax of immaterial abstraction and material consumption,' except that today this parallax does not simply signify the 'crisscrossing between the extremes of spectacular finance and world-historical shopping.'[89] Rather, it designates the veritable crisscrossing between a double-faced immaterial abstraction—both value and spirit, capital and metaphysics/religion—and empirical life—in which capital makes a second reappearance as the Master. The result of this has so far been that the posthuman subject–object lives in the crisscrossing between an insatiable craving for immortality, which can be fulfilled by shopping and killing the externalized projection of its past pre-posthuman—also known as mortal human. Is this all that can come after the subject?

Recapitulating, and Slightly Beyond

According to my line of argument, what comes after the subject is the subject–object of commodity fetishism, which has virtually existed since the inception of secular capitalist modernity, yet has gradually actualized historically and reached its full-fledged and self-conscious actualization in postmodernism. Prior to this latter stage, conceptions of subjectivity as transcendent to the object prevailed in the discourse of secular capitalist modernity, while also sustaining the corollary conception of power as embodied in a transcendent State that controls its subjects by means of ideology. The shift to the self-conscious–actualization of the subject–object is paralleled by the shift from State and ideology to the market and biopower/biopolitics.

Nevertheless, by considering the capitalist commodification of labor-power and by examining the modes of temporality reappropriated and/or introduced by the capitalist mode of production, we come to see that current conceptualizations of biopower as a power, the object of which is the administration of the biological body, are obsolete. Rather, the condition of commodity fetishism eventually leads to a biopolitics that regulates the subject–object's relationship to two competing modes of temporality. On the one hand, the age-old concept of eternity—insofar as, with capitalism, the body matters exclusively as the bearer of labor-power, which is potentiality and with a mode of temporality that is eternity—and, on the other hand, the radically new temporality introduced by capitalism through surplus-value (i.e., infinite diachrony). The latter, however, is a mode of temporality that pertains only to the virtual level and can never be actualized—the actual always has a finite duration. Nevertheless, this virtual temporality has two major effects on the actual.

First, it renders actual enjoyment impossible, and thereby transforms it into surplus-enjoyment—the perpetual yearning for evermore enjoyment, or enjoyment in excess. Second, it imbues the unconscious with the illusory certainty of the immortality of the actual, which is to say, the immortality of biological bodies, as the secular fantasy of immortality that takes hold eventually in postmodernism. At this stage, biopower lures subjects–objects to cede their eternity for the sake of living in (an imagined) infinite diachrony. This fantasy is sustained through two major sacrificial mechanisms.

On the one hand, an incessant and insatiable consumerism, during which subject–objects strive neither for actual enjoyment nor for monetary or other practical and/or utilitarian profit, as moments of crisis and debt make clear, but for the sustenance of the infinite duration of the durable—that is, of their (illusion of) immortality. On the other hand, given that immortality now becomes the sole feature based on which subject–objects can still maintain the old cherished illusion of a humanity that transcends its counterparts (e.g., from animals, plants, and inanimate objects to those humans perceived as subhumans), bioracism emerges as a further sacrificial practice that, as is always the case with racism, is misconstrued as a means for self-preservation. Biopolitics divides what must live from what must die by fostering a break between the superrace of the immortals and what this same race constructs as the subrace of the mortals; that is, as those who do not strive for surplus-enjoyment and the immortality of the actual but rather indulge in actual enjoyment and in the death of the actual.

Finally, one further capitalist appropriation of eternity deserves a brief mention here. Being the temporality of the Real, of course eternity cannot be experienced empirically; it can only be yearned for asymptotically. Yet, a fake or imitation eternity is supplied through what Lacan calls 'imitation surplus *jouissance* [*semblant de plus-de-jouir*]'—that is, 'the homogeneous equivalent of whatever surplus *jouissance* is produced by our industry' of the '"[c]onsumer society."'[90] This imitation jouissance consists in distraction, insofar as it makes one forget one's (empirical and historical) diachrony, which is the empirical state closest to experiencing something like eternity.

As we know from the work of Émile Durkheim, Marcel Mauss, and George Bataille, this was the function of archaic and pagan religious festivals, those ecstatic 'lacunae' that interrupted the linear time of purposeful and socially productive activity, of which the later religious rituals of various monotheisms were residues. In today's society, however, the sources of such distraction are ubiquitous and incessant, ranging from mass communication and entertainment media, addictive substances, and work-alcoholism, to consumerism, entertainment, working out, and sports. It is for this reason that, as Benjamin astutely discerned:

> Capitalism is the celebration of a cult *sans rêve et sans merci* [without dream or mercy (i.e., without a break)]. There are no 'weekdays.' There is no day that is not a feast day, in the terrible sense that all its sacred pomp is unfolded before us; each day commands the utter fealty of each worshiper.[91]

Moreover, in Benjamin's admirable insight, capitalism is 'not a formation conditioned by religion,' as in Max Weber, but 'an essentially religious phenomenon' that, nevertheless, differs from *all* other religions in four respects.[92] The first, as we just saw, lies in its 'permanence of the cult'; the second lies in the fact that 'capitalism is a purely cultic religion'—that is, it 'has no specific body of dogma, no theology,' except of course for 'utilitarianism,' which here 'acquires…religious overtones.' Third, 'capitalism is probably the first instance of a cult that creates guilt, not atonement'; in fact it 'makes guilt pervasive,' as 'a vast sense of guilt that is unable to find relief seizes on the cult, not to atone for this guilt but to make it universal.' Fourth, in 'the religion of capitalism…its God must be hidden from it,' which is why 'what has been repressed…is capital itself, which pays interest on the hell of the unconscious.'[93]

What this chapter has shown is a fifth difference between capitalism and all other religions. In capitalism's permanent cult of universal guilt where God is unconscious, eternity and infinity overlap and both are available in the market—that is, in all our waking and sleeping life. As for whether anything else can come after the subject, this is a matter that hinges on the temporalities that are constitutive of both economy and subjectivity.

Notes

1. My position here deviates to some extent from Étienne Balibar's reading of Marx's relation among the components of the labor process in industrial or machinized production. The 'labour process' in general consists of (1) the 'personal activity' of 'labour'; (2) the 'object of labour'; and (3) the 'means of labour' (Louis Althusser and Étienne Balibar, *Reading Capital* (London: Verso, 2009: 270–271). The difference between the eras of handicraft (and manufacturing) and industrial production consists in a transformation of the form in which the three elements of labor combine. Handicrafts rely on a '"*technique*"' as '*the indissoluble ensemble* of a means of labour or tool, *and a worker*, moulded to its use by apprenticeship and habit,' just as the tool must itself 'be adapted to the human organism' (Althusser and Balibar, p. 267). With the introduction of the industrial 'machine-tool' this 'relationship is inverted' so that the human 'organism must adapt itself to the instrument' (Althusser and Balibar, p. 268). From this Balibar infers that the 'machine-tool makes the organization of production completely independent of the characteristics of human labour-power: at the same stroke, the means of the labour and the labourer are completely separated and acquire different forms of development' (Ibid.). But if the laborer's organism must adapt itself to the instrument, then what takes place here is not a separation between labor and means of labor but rather the subjugation of the former by the latter. Thus, the elements constituting machinic production are indeed restructured around '*the unity of the means…and the object of labour*,' under which the labor activity (and the laborer) is entirely subordinated—rather than being simply separated (Ibid.). It is because this total subordination of the labor to the means of labor eliminates the individual character of the laborer's 'technique' that a unit of production no longer consists of a particular group of specialized laborers but is rather a 'material skeleton independent of the labourers themselves' (*Capital, Vol. 1*)—a 'set of fixed machines ready to receive any workers' (Ibid.).

2. Jacques Lacan, *The Four Fundamental Concepts of Psychoanalysis*, ed. Jacques-Alain Miller. Trans. Alan Sheridan (New York: W. W. Norton, 1981), p. 62.
3. Karl Marx, *Capital: A Critique of Political Economy, Vol. 1*. Trans. Ben Fowkes (London: Penguin Books, 1990), pp. 164–165.
4. Ibid., pp. 165–166.
5. Étienne Balibar, *The Philosophy of Marx*. Trans. Chris Turner (London: Verso, 2007): p. 58; Georg Simmel, *The Philosophy of Money*, 2nd ed., ed. David Frisby. Trans. Tom Bottomore and David Frisby from a first draft by Kaethe Mengelberg (London: Routledge, 1990): pp. 148, 152.
6. Marx (1990), pp. 164–165.
7. Balibar (2007), pp. 58–59.
8. Ibid., pp. 56, 64–65.
9. Ibid., p. 67.
10. Alexandre Kojève, *Introduction to the Reading of Hegel: Lectures on the Phenomenology of Spirit*, assemb. Raymond Queneau, ed. Allan Bloom, trans. James H. Nichols, Jr. (Ithaca: Cornell University Press, 1980), p. 25.
11. By referring to 'stages' I do not imply a teleological conception of history of the Hegelian type, but rather I mean to acknowledge the fact that, following Spinoza, the essence and attributes of substance strive for their maximum actualization within historical time, and it is these different degrees of actualization that my term 'stages' indicates. If there is any *telos* in history, this is the maximum actualization of the potential (essence) of substance, and whatever of this potential is not yet actualized at any given historical moment, nevertheless, exists, albeit only virtually, as part of the essence of substance. This is why one can know the essence of substance in its entirety only retroactively, after its full actualization—which is why the self-consciousness of humanity *qua* posthumanity could not emerge but after a considerable actualization of commodity fetishism.
12. Balibar (2007), p. 76.
13. Ibid., pp. 77–78.
14. Ibid., p. 78. This is why, as Balibar remarks, Marx's 'theory of fetishism' is 'one of the greatest theoretical constructions of modern philosophy,' as it shows 'that there is no theory of objectivity without a theory of subjectivity. *By rethinking the constitution of social objectivity, Marx at the same time virtually revolutionized the concept of the "subject"*' (Balibar, pp. 56,

64–65) as precisely the subject-object. Through the concept of commodity fetishism Marx overcame both the dualism between subject and object and that between transcendence and immanence.

15. Ibid., pp. 76–77.
16. Michel Foucault, 'The Subject and Power,' in Brian Wallis (ed.), *Art After Modernism: Rethinking Representation* (New York/Boston: The New Museum of Contemporary Art and David R. Godine, 1999), p. 420.
17. Baruch/Benedict de Spinoza, *The Collected Works of Spinoza*, 'part I, prop. 18 and part. 2, prop. 43, schol.' Ed. and trans. Edwin Curley (Princeton: Princeton University Press, 1985), p. 479.
18. Given that, according to Spinoza, there is only one substance, the reader might wonder how one can treat one specific historical object or era, secular capitalist modernity, as if it were tantamount to substance, since there have been various other historical eras. In other parts of my work I explain how each historical era is a specific modification of one and the same substance, which then must actualize itself in its own stages. See also Kordela *Capital: At Least It Kills Time (Spinoza, Marx, Lacan, and Temporality)* and *Rethinking Marxism* 18(4), pp. 539–563 (Kordela, 2006, 2013).
19. Marx (1990), p. 165.
20. Balibar (2007), p. 66.
21. Marx (1990), p. 255.
22. Balibar (2007), p. 67.
23. Furthermore, as I argue elsewhere, power has always been biopower, since the formation of the most archaic societies and is not only a form of power specific to the capitalist mode of production. Nevertheless, there are substantial historical modifications of biopower that clearly distinguish its forms in each era, depending on both the era's mode of production and its epistemological configuration of the relation between immanence and transcendence. See Kordela, Biopolitics: From Tribes to Commodity Fetishism, *Differences* 24:1.
24. Foucault, *The History of Sexuality. Volume 1: An Introduction*. Trans. Robert Hurley (New York: Vintage Books, 1990): pp. 136–140.
25. Giorgio Agamben, *Homo Sacer: Sovereign Power and Bare Life*. Trans. Daniel Heller-Roazen (Stanford: Stanford Univeristy Press, 1998), pp. 127–129.
26. Agamben (1998), p. 114.
27. Ibid., pp. 124, 119, 73.

28. Ibid., p. 176.
29. Marx, *Grundrisse: Foundations of the Critique of Political Economy (Rough Draft)*. Trans. Martin Nicolaus (London: Penguin Books and *New Left Review*, 1993), p. 267.
30. Paolo Virno, *A Grammar of the Multitude: For an Analysis of Contemporary Forms of Life*. Trans. Isabella Bertoletti, James Cascaito, and Andrea Casson (Los Angeles: Semiotext(e), 2004), p. 82.
31. Ibid.
32. Ibid.
33. Foucault (1990), p. 136; Foucault, *Society Must Be Defended: Lectures at the Collège de France, 1975–1976,* trans. David Macey (New York: Picador, 2003), p. 259.
34. Ibid., p. 127.
35. Spinoza (1985), 'pt. 4, preface,' p. 544.
36. Spinoza, *Ethics* (1985), 'part II, prop. 44, cor. 2, dem.,' p. 481.
37. Gilles Deleuze, *Spinoza: Practical Philosophy*. Trans. Robert Hurley (San Francisco: City Lights Books, 1988), p. 62.
38. Ibid.
39. Ibid.
40. Spinoza (1985), 'part V, prop. 29,' pp. 609–610.
41. See Jacques Lacan, *Book XVII. The Other Side of Psychoanalysis*, ed. Jacques-Alain Miller, trans. Russell Grigg (New York: W. W. Norton, 2007).
42. Marx (1990), p. 138.
43. Ferdinand de Saussure, *Course in General Linguistics*, ed. Charles Bally et al., trans. Roy Harris (London: Duckworth, 1966), p. 115.
44. Ibid., p. 69.
45. Foucault, *The Order of Things: An Archaeology of the Human Sciences* (New York: Vintage, 1970), p. 42.
46. Marx (1993), pp. 663, 659.
47. Marx (1990), p. 257.
48. Éric Alliez, *Capital Times: Tales from the Conquest of Time*, Foreword by Gilles Deleuze, trans. Georges Van Den Abbeele (Minneapolis: University of Minnesota Press, 1996),: p. 7.
49. Aristotle, *The Politics*, trans. T. A. Sinclair, revised by Trevor J. Saunders (London: Penguin Books, 1992), p. 81; 1256b40.
50. Ibid., pp. 82–83, 84; 1256b40, 1257b10.
51. Ibid., p. 84; 1257b25.

52. Marx (1990), p. 253.
53. Aristotle (1992), p. 84; 1257b25.
54. Marx (1990), pp. 253, 251.
55. Aristotle (1992), pp. 84–85; 1257b25–40.
56. Ibid.
57. Deleuze, Postscript on Control Societies. In *Negotiations, 1972–1990*, trans. Martin Joughin (New York: Columbia University Press, 1995), p. 191.
58. Richard Dienst, *The Bonds of Debt: Borrowing Against the Common Good* (London: Verso, 2011), p. 179.
59. Ibid., p. 166.
60. Ibid., citing Walter Benjamin, *Gesammelte Schriften* (Frankfurt: Suhrkamp, 1972–1989), 1/3 1,240.
61. Dienst (2011), p. 129.
62. Ibid.
63. Ibid., p. 124.
64. Ibid.
65. Deleuze, How Do We Recognize Structuralism? Trans. Melissa McMahon and Charles J. Stivale. In *Desert Islands and Other Texts 1953–1974*, ed. David Lapoujade (Los Angeles: Semiotext(e), 2004), pp. 170–192.
66. The 'individual' makes its last appearance (i.e., still functions as an operative category) in modernism, that is, until the end of the disciplinary society. This is Deleuze's point when, in the same text that greatly inspired Dienst, he writes: 'Disciplinary societies have two poles: signatures standing for *individuals*, and numbers or places in a register standing for their position in a *mass*.…[The] power [of disciplines] both amasses and individuates, that is, it fashions those over whom it's exerted into a body of people and molds the individuality of each member of that body.…In control societies, on the other hand, the key thing is no longer a signature or number but a code.…The digital language of control is made up of codes indicating whether access to some information should be allowed or denied. We're no longer dealing with a duality of mass and individual. Individuals become "*dividuals*," and masses become samples, data, markets, or "*banks*"' (Deleuze 1995, pp. 179–180).
67. Dienst (2011), p. 124.
68. Georges Bataille, *Theory of Religion*. Trans. Robert Hurley (New York: Zone Books, 1989): pp. 32–33.

69. Ibid., p. 33; emphasis mine.
70. Ibid., p. 34.
71. Ibid., pp. 33, 17–19.
72. Ibid., p. 35.
73. Ibid., p. 37.
74. Ibid., p. 38.
75. Ibid.
76. Ibid., p. 43.
77. Ibid., p. 44.
78. Ibid., pp. 34–35.
79. Ibid., p. 35.
80. Marx (1990), pp. 165, 167.
81. Dienst (2011), p. 124.
82. Lacan (1981), p. 59.
83. Dienst (2011), pp. 124–125.
84. Ibid., pp. 128–129; referring to *Harvard Design School Guide to Shopping*, eds. Chuihua Judy Chung, Jeffrey Inaba, Rem Koolhaas, Sze Tsung Leon (Köln: Taschen, 2001), p. 51.
85. Foucault (2003), p. 254.
86. Ibid., pp. 59–60, 255–257.
87. Ibid., p. 61.
88. Ibid.
89. Dienst (2011), p. 125.
90. Lacan (2007), pp. 80–81.
91. Walter Benjamin, Capitalism as Religion. In *Selected Writings, Vol.1, 1913–1926*, trans. Rodney Livingstone (Cambridge: Belknap/Harvard Press, 1996, p. 288; second set of brackets inserted by me).
92. Ibid.
93. Ibid.

Bibliography

Agamben, Giorgio. 1998. *Homo Sacer: Sovereign Power and Bare Life*. Trans. Daniel Heller-Roazen. Stanford: Stanford Univeristy Press.

Alliez, Éric. 1996. *Capital Times: Tales from the Conquest of Time*. Foreword by Gilles Deleuze. Trans. Georges Van Den Abbeele. Minneapolis: University of Minnesota Press.

Althusser, Louis, and Étienne Balibar. 2009. *Reading Capital.* London: Verso.
Aristotle. 1992. *The Politics.* Trans. T. A. Sinclair. Revised by Trevor J. Saunders. London: Penguin Books.
Balibar, Étienne. 2007. *The Philosophy of Marx.* Trans. Chris Turner. London: Verso.
Bataille, Georges. 1989. *Theory of Religion.* Trans. Robert Hurley. New York: Zone Books.
Benjamin, Walter. 1972–1989. *Gesammelte Schriften.* Frankfurt: Suhrkamp.
———. 1996. Capitalism as Religion. In *Selected Writings Vol. 1, 1913–1926.* Trans. Rodney Livingstone, 288–291. Cambridge: Belknap/Harvard Press.
Chung, Chuihua Judy, Jeffrey Inaba, Rem Koolhaas, and Sze Tsung Leon, eds. 2001. *Harvard Design School Guide to Shopping.* Köln: Taschen.
de Saussure, Ferdinand. 1966. *Course in General Linguistics,* ed. Charles Bally, et al. Trans. Roy Harris. London: Duckworth.
Deleuze, Gilles. 1988. *Spinoza: Practical Philosophy.* Trans. Robert Hurley. San Francisco: City Lights Books.
———. 1995. Postscript on Control Societies. In *Negotiations, 1972–1990.* Trans. Martin Joughin, 177–180. New York: Columbia University Press.
———. 2004. How Do We Recognize Structuralism? Trans. Melissa McMahon and Charles J. Stivale. In *Desert Islands and Other Texts 1953–1974,* ed. David Lapoujade, pp. 170–192. Los Angeles: Semiotext(e).
Dienst, Richard. 2011. *The Bonds of Debt: Borrowing Against the Common Good.* London: Verso.
Foucault, Michel. 1970. *The Order of Things: An Archaeology of the Human Sciences.* New York: Vintage.
———. 1990. *The History of Sexuality. Volume 1: An Introduction.* Trans. Robert Hurley. New York: Vintage Books.
———. 1999. The Subject and Power. In *Art After Modernism: Rethinking Representation,* ed. Brian Wallis, 417–432. New York/Boston: The New Museum of Contemporary Art and David R. Godine.
———. 2003. *Society Must Be Defended: Lectures at the Collège de France, 1975–1976.* Trans. David Macey. New York: Picador.
Kojève, Alexandre. 1980. *Introduction to the Reading of Hegel: Lectures on the Phenomenology of Spirit.* Assemb. Raymond Queneau, ed. Allan Bloom. Trans. James H. Nichols, Jr. Ithaca: Cornell University Press.
Kordela, A. Kiarina. 2006. Capital: At Least It Kills Time (Spinoza, Marx, Lacan, and Temporality). *Rethinking Marxism* 18 (4): 539–563.
———. 2013. *Being, Time, Bios: Capitalism and Ontology.* Albany: SUNY Press.

———. 2014. Biopolitics: From Tribes to Commodity Fetishism. *Differences* 24: 1.

Lacan, Jacques. 1981. *The Four Fundamental Concepts of Psychoanalysis,* ed. Jacques-Alain Miller. Trans. Alan Sheridan. New York: W. W. Norton.

———. 1991. In *Le Séminaire. Livre XVII: L'envers de la Psychanalyse, 1969–1970,* ed. Jacques-Alain Miller. Paris: Seuil.

———. 2007. *Book XVII. The Other Side of Psychoanalysis,* ed. Jacques-Alain Miller. Trans. Russell Grigg. New York: W. W. Norton.

Marx, Karl. 1990. *Capital: A Critique of Political Economy, Vol. 1.* Trans. Ben Fowkes. London: Penguin Books.

———. 1993. Grundrisse: Foundations of the Critique of Political Economy (Rough Draft). Trans. Martin Nicolaus. London: Penguin Books/New Left Review.

Simmel, Georg. 1990. *The Philosophy of Money,* 2nd ed., ed. David Frisby. Trans. Tom Bottomore and David Frisby from a first draft by Kaethe Mengelberg. London: Routledge.

Spinoza, Baruch/Benedict de. 1985. *The Collected Works of Spinoza.* Ed. and trans. Edwin Curley. Princeton: Princeton University Press.

Virno, Paolo. 2004. *A Grammar of the Multitude: For an Analysis of Contemporary Forms of Life.* Trans. Isabella Bertoletti, James Cascaito, and Andrea Casson. Los Angeles: Semiotext(e).

L'extermination de tout Symbolisme des Cieux: Reading the Lacanian *Letter* as Inhuman 'Apparatus' and Its Implications for Ecological Thinking

Kevin Andrew Spicer

Toward the very end of Sean McGrath's essay, 'The Question Concerning Nature,' he notes the very common dismissal of an overly pious reading of Heidegger's notion of *Gelassenheit*. Canvassing the 'Ecology without Nature' (EWN) philosophy of Timothy Morton, McGrath alludes to the problem with the 'green' reading of Heidegger that argues *Gelassenheit* leaves one bereft of political discernment, placidly accepting 'the way things are: Should we also let the BP oil spill be? Should we let the decimation of the Amazon rainforest be?'[1] McGrath correctly notes that this is a slight misreading of Heidegger, as '*Gelassenheit* was never offered as a method of environmental practice; it is, rather, an undermining of techno-scientific-capitalist thought itself, an overturning of its basic assumption, that the human is or ought to be the master of time.'[2]

Requiring *Gelassenheit* to become a method 'is to leave the will to mastery at the root of our crisis unchallenged.' According to McGrath, 'Morton's mistake is to assume that a contemplative approach to the question concerning nature has been tried and found wanting. On the

K.A. Spicer (✉)
University of St. Francis, Joliet, IL, USA

G. Basu Thakur, J.M. Dickstein (eds.), *Lacan and the Nonhuman*,
The Palgrave Lacan Series, DOI 10.1007/978-3-319-63817-1_5

contrary, it has been found wanting without ever being tried.' When one switches registers a bit to ask about Lacan's usefulness for the ecocritical and environmental philosophies of the late twentieth and early twenty-first centuries, one cannot help but think something identical has happened to his thought: numerous scholars have, as I hope to show, 'found it wanting without ever really trying [it] yet.'

There has been no small quantity of ink spilled showing that Lacan's work will not really help one talk about the nonhuman at all. His thought is just another exemplary case of 'structural linguistic correlationism' (Johnston)[3]; a typical anthropocentric humanist who cannot think the nature of the animal (Derrida); or, perhaps worst of all, a scatological thinker whose worry about what humans will do with their 'shit' keeps him from articulating the 'ecological thought' so necessary today in the Anthropocene (Morton).[4] Hoping to steer clear of all these criticisms, I would like to argue that understanding how ecological thinking is itself split between ecology as both a science and a philosophical regime within the humanities opens up a path that can capitalize on Lacan's views on science and mathematical symbolism and formalism.[5]

It is Lacan's focus on the 'letter in the Real'—not the 'matheme,' nor the Signifier—that allows a fruitful understanding of the fundamentally traumatic kernel of the ecological Real. Grasping how the letter in Lacan's treatment of science—which should be connected to the recent work of Mackenzie Wark on the 'apparatus'—gives one access to the nonhuman nature of reality clearly demonstrates the potential usefulness of Lacanian psychoanalysis for continuing current ecological philosophy's focus on the decentering of anthropocentric thought.

Almost 30 years ago now, the philosopher and media theorist, Vilém Flusser, composed an essay entitled 'Orders of Magnitude and Humanism,' wherein he quite clearly and parsimoniously described how humanity's scientific progress since the age of the Greeks has exploded awareness of diverse 'orders of magnitude.'[6] Flusser noted that it was 'easy for the ancients to say,' as Protagoras did, that 'man is the measure of all things' (p. 160). Truly, '[t]hen everything in the world could indeed be measured in centimeters, hours, dollars (or the contemporary equivalents thereof). What was not measurable thus was unmeasurable' (Ibid). Nevertheless, after the invention of the lens, which allows one not only to see the incredibly distant but also the miniscule, awareness of different 'orders of magnitude' in reality becomes much more salient.

The explosion proliferates so quickly that Flusser fittingly notes that it would not have been enough for the Church to destroy all of Galileo's work—the 'penetration would not have been avoided.'

> For the world has not only expanded into space in order to bend at one of its horizons and to fray into quarks at the other, it has also expanded into time, in order to creep into the [B]ig [B]ang on the one hand, and into the quantum leap on the other. It would have been necessary to burn the stop-watches too.[7]

The inability to keep all these different orders straight results in a complete breakdown of the anthropocentric, humanist perspective, according to Flusser:

> Besides, the world has also expanded with respect to values, thereby assuming inhuman dimensions, in gross net products on the one hand, and calculations of cost on the other. The slide rules would have had to be burned too. In short: man has advanced into the inhuman, the inhuman strikes back at him, and under these blows, humanism breaks down.[8]

In this very short essay, Flusser says that one's understanding of these various orders of magnitude call for '[a] Ptolemaic counterrevolution,' a 'completely new humanism' that would 'call attention to the priority of the human order of magnitude.'[9] Flusser in his essay suggests—incredibly aphoristically—that it is impossible to put the genie back in the bottle.

Given that the bottle has already been opened, it behooves us, asserts Flusser, to be attentive to the ways in which we switch between these different orders of magnitude we have come to know:

> The new humanism cannot want to deny that different orders of measurement overlap each other and interpenetrate. On the contrary, it has to emphasize that, for each order of magnitude, there is a typical epistemology, ethics, and aesthetics that is effective, and that, in spite of the gray zones, abysses gape between the orders of magnitude. Thus, it is mischief to apply the geometry of what is perceptible by the senses to the astronomical

order of magnitude or causal thinking to the order of magnitude of particles of atom nuclei. The specificity of each order of magnitude would have to enable the new humanism to call attention to the priority of the human order of magnitude.[10]

Now, it is perfectly possible to wonder about this bid for a 'new *humanism*,' and a redoubled effort to 'pay attention to the priority of the *human* order of magnitude.' After all, things like exponential notation and transfinite arithmetic allow us to *think* and *calculate* phenomena that so escape the terrestrial senses that they are impossible to actually picture, let alone fully understand.[11]

This is not even to mention that we have been using these tools for a really long time—exponentiation goes back to Descartes and both scientific notation and Cantor's work on transfinite arithmetic are now well over a hundred years old. Today it seems even more necessary to think intensely about the sheer uncanniness that comes through the knowledge of everything from quantum mechanical systems to the existence of gravitational waves. Flusser is right to say that awareness of differing orders of magnitude require certain 'effective theories': using Newton's Laws will not be helpful to us on the subatomic order of magnitude; employing notions of space–time manifolds 'to the production of ink pens would be stupid.'[12]

As helpful as Flusser's short remarks are, there appear to be two different kinds of prostheses in the essay. The first comes through the variety of technological inventions (e.g., the lens, the telescope, the microscope, the slide rule, etc.), whereas the second includes the slightly more abstract (though no less material) mathematical tools (e.g., scientific notation, mathematical formulas, etc.). It is the latter that needs a theorization through a Lacanian lens.

Although Lacan does not himself have any full-fledged history of science—relying, instead, largely on the work of Alexandre Koyré—he does have a great deal to say about the kind of subject that has been birthed by modern science. What is most useful in Lacan's work is his awareness of the substantially destabilizing and fundamentally traumatic nature of scientific knowledge; this is, a knowledge that, at the end of the day, puts to the sword many humanist perspectives, making them ultimately 'superfluous.'[13] Of course, Koyré and Lacan were certainly by no means the only ones to see this.

The extreme gap between the sciences and the humanities shows up in extremely clear ways (e.g., in Hannah Arendt's *The Human Condition*). In the Prologue to this text, Arendt notes the profound splitting of our knowledge, especially of the subatomic world, evidenced clearly by her mention of Erwin Schrödinger:

> The trouble concerns the facts that the 'truths' of the modern scientific world view, though they can be demonstrated in mathematical formulas and proved technologically, will no longer lend themselves to normal expression in speech and thought. The moment these 'truths' are spoken of conceptually and coherently, the resulting statements will be 'not perhaps as meaningless as a "triangular circle," but much more so than a "winged lion"' (Erwin Schrödinger). ...For the sciences today have been forced to adopt a 'language' of mathematical symbols which, though it was originally meant only as an abbreviation for spoken statements, now contains statements that in no way can be translated back into speech. ...[Scientists] move in a world where speech has lost its power.[14]

Given that there is very little doubt as to the accuracy of these statements, Koyré and Lacan argue that something similar was already at work much earlier in history, going back, ultimately, to the first great humiliators of human specialness—Copernicus and Kepler.

In a 1959 essay on Ernest Jones, Lacan discusses the monumental sea-change that occurs not solely when we figured out that the Earth was not the center of the Universe (Ancient sources had already floated such ideas around, to be sure), but also when we began to use the formalism of mathematical language to model and describe the 'heavenly spheres'; Lacan argues that the history of science:

> ...brilliantly demonstrates, in the birth of the theory of gravitation, that it was only on the basis of the extermination of all symbolism of the heavens [*l'extermination de tout symbolisme des cieux*] that the terrestrial foundations of modern physics could be established—namely, that as long as some requirement to ascribe to the heavenly orbits a 'perfect' shape was maintained (insofar as it implied, for example, the circle's preeminence over the

ellipse) from Giordano Bruno to Kepler and from Kepler to Newton, it thwarted the developed of the theory's key equations.[15]

Lacan's language pulls no punches here—describing the heavenly spheres with mathematics requires '*l'extermination de tout symbolisme des cieux*'; freed from the necessity for the planets to match the 'perfect' shape of the circle, we made them no longer heavenly at all. Moreover, nothing makes our 'humanist references more superfluous' than grasping science's ability to bypass the capture of the Imaginary.[16] Asking the world always to submit itself to humanism—as our Imaginary relations to the world so often do—makes it clear why Jean-Claude Milner is perfectly correct to say that '[t]he Imaginary as such is radically foreign to modern science.'[17]

My intervention here with regard to this 'extermination of all symbolism of the heavens' takes its cue from a couple of different angles, many of them very familiar to Lacanians. The first is Tom Eyers's attempt at a rapprochement between Lacanian psychoanalysis and current object-oriented ontology (OOO) forms of philosophy in his 'Lacanian Materialism and the Question of the Real.'[18] Eyers's article argues that if one grasps the way in which the *letter* in Lacan is of the Real while the Signifier is that of the Symbolic, this opens up the possibility for a discussion of certain 'non-human agenc[ies]' that have become the main theoretical objects of so many of the new speculative realisms. Eyers quite rightly argues that 'when we question the supposed inextricability of language from the world, the symmetry of a human/non-human topography, offers a complementary discourse centred on those aspects of existence that slip between binaries of human and non-human, life and death, material and ideal.'[19]

Following Lacan's definition of the 'letter' in 'The Instance of the Letter in the Unconscious' as 'the material medium [*support*] that concrete language borrows from discourse,'[20] Eyers proposes the counterargument that Lacan is hardly guilty of being 'a covert linguistic idealist,' as Nancy, Lacoue-Labarthe, and Derrida all argued. Instead, for Eyers, these critiques of Lacan all force one to 'ask whether their argument takes full cognisance of this paradoxical materiality of the signifier, its shrinking away from, and disruption of subjectivity.'[21] At times, Eyers argues for a reading that sees the letter as itself just a split within the Signifier; thus, for Lacan, there are 'two levels of discourse—that is, the isolated letter or signifier-in-isolation, extracted from the relations of negative reference that ultimately give meaning to language. ...'[22] For the purposes this chapter, it is most helpful to go to a couple of later Lacanian texts to ferret out the idea of the 'letter in the Real' as quite terminologically distinct from speaking of this very same letter as a 'signifier-in-isolation.'

Dany Nobus's reading of Lacan's later work on Joyce and also the key essay, 'Lituraterre,' lays out with great clarity Lacan's insistence that '[w]hereas the signifier is situated within the Symbolic, the letter belongs to the Real.'[23] Even though Nobus's reading focuses on the letter in the Real as it relates to literature and the work of Joyce, there is a way to see very similar functions in terms of mathematics and science and the aforementioned extermination of all heavenly symbolism. Nobus's utilization of natural languages as the example for understanding the Lacanian letter is simple enough: 'When Lacan claimed that letters belong to the Real, he intimated that as phonograms they are completely stripped of all meaning; it is impossible to say what the letter "X" means, because as a phonogram it does not have any meaning whatsoever.'[24]

Nobus also is correct to notice a strong consistency in Lacan's thinking:

> Now, some fifteen years later [after 'The Purloined Letter'], Lacan surmises that the letter cannot sustain itself as such within the Symbolic order when it is radically deprived of meaning. Formerly the signifier *par excellence*, an essentially meaningless unit, the letter now presents itself as a radical anti-signifier, an excrement that has turned against its own progenitor.[25]

Nobus's choice of the example, in the letter 'X' is coincidentally very fruitful for a discussion of how all of this relates not just to literature but also to mathematics and mathematical language. In a couple of spots in Lacan's Seminar XIV, he has recourse to Bertrand Russell's description of mathematicians' use of formulas and terms in ways that nobody knows what they are talking about 'nor whether what we are saying has the slightest truth.'[26]

Granting that all of this is no doubt old hat for Lacanians, scholars outside of psychoanalytic circles have recently taken up this focus on the letter in the Real as well. Exemplary is Noah Horowitz's recent work, which provides even more support for arguing that Lacanian thought provides a great deal of material for understanding how exactly this 'extermination of all symbolism of the heavens' functions precisely in terms of mathematics and science. Horowitz's project in his two major texts—*Reality in the Name of God, or Divine Insistence* and *Divine Name Verification*—is admittedly rather different from this chapter's; there are several key ideas regarding the notion of the Lacanian letter that are useful here.

The texts by Horowitz should be read as instances of healthy caution toward the OOO and speculative realism (SR) movements away from the linguistic turn; instead of simply agreeing with Barad and others that we have given too much power to language,[27] Horowitz's two books double-down on the irreducibility of this very same linguistic turn (broadening this adjective, of course, to include things like the Lacanian letter).[28] His gamble relies a great deal—though it would seem not be that big a gamble for Lacanians as Horowitz's interpretation accurately reproduces the readings of Eyers and Nobus—on Lacan's placing of the *letter* within the register of the Real: '…Lacan relegates letters to the register of the Real rather than to the Symbolic. The letters are excluded from symbolization for Lacan.'[29]

Horowitz continues on to say that this focus on the letter becomes clearest when Lacan speaks of the texts of science and mathematics as he did earlier in the citations from Seminar XIV, for these texts 'are composed of formulas, equations, etc. consisting almost exclusively of numbers and letters.'[30] Following an essay by Tzahi Weiss, Horowitz asserts:

> [T]hese letters are not signifiers, but the 'material structure that creates the possibility of the signifier' itself. Letters have 'no referent' outside the register of signification itself. Since meaning is ideal, the letter is identified with materiality. And this material is opaque and resistant, but insistent insofar as it can destroy meaning. But it is not the materiality of the ink on paper. It is of the Real, which means it always returns to its place, is impossibility, and names the gaps or fractures of meaningful networks.[31]

Horowitz's keen awareness that '[f]or Lacan also, one can overcome fantasy precisely by turning to math and its way of reducing reality to letters. …'[32] Even though Horowitz does not cite the key passage cited earlier from the essay on Ernest Jones's symbolism—nor does he put it in exactly the same language as that of Nobus's description of the letter as an 'anti-signifier'; however, he does grasp how this all resonates with Lacan's conception of modern science as 'becom[ing] possible once the real was reduced to the mathematical and that means to letters. Science thereby devotes itself to an analysis of purely differential being. It *literalizes reality* such that it can see it as diverse and multiple.'[33] It is exactly this upsetting of Imaginary–anthropocentric meaning that seems most appropriate for synthesizing with the nonhuman turn.

So many Lacanian discoveries fan out to connect with numerous posthumanist arguments—all starting from the mingling of the letter in the Real (seen through mathematical formalism), the importance of writing, and ultimately with the description of this very same Real as what *never stops writing itself*, or as the impossible itself.[34] Cary Wolfe's argument, for instance, in his now-canonical *What Is Posthumanism?* concerning the prosthetic nature of *writing* is thoroughly consistent with Lacanian thought. Wolfe's attempt to show an agreement between systems theory and deconstruction relies heavily not only on this idea of *prosthesis* but also on the fundamentally inhuman nature of this apparatus.

Wolfe mentions on several different occasions how both Derrida and Luhmann allow one to think of *writing* as itself a prosthesis of/for the human being. *Writing* is something that clues one into the fact that 'the human is, at its core and in its very constitution, radically ahuman and constitutively prosthetic.'[35] Wolfe's summary of the Derridean distinction between the obsession with the auto-affection of the voice and the privileging of speech is itself shown through the *grammè* of writing, which is defined as 'a recursive domain of iterative communication that is, properly understood, *fundamentally ahuman or even antihuman*.'[36]

In the interests of investigating a bit more closely this idea of the prosthesis in Wolfe and of its potential connections with discussions of the nonhuman, we should begin by thinking through the tools of mathematics and science—the letter in the Real for Lacan—as themselves prostheses. Despite Johnston's argument that Lacan's work suffers from a problematic overreliance on the 'pure' sciences (as opposed to the life sciences of biology, and so on), it is this focus on the letter in the Real that shows a path toward the nonhuman that travels along the fundamental *inhumanity* of mathematics and science.[37] Given the understanding that the letter is relegated to the Real, we can easily see some connections with contemporary advocates of rethinking the human's connection to nonhuman reality; Mackenzie Wark's recent text, *Molecular Red*, comes to mind most readily.

In this text, which does not utilize nor even mention the psychoanalytic tradition, Wark notes something identical to Lacan; when science goes to the extreme limits of reality and knowledge, it becomes clear that:

> ...[t]here is something inhuman about science. Its modes of perception, modeling and verifying are outside the parameters of the human sensorium, even though they are dependent on an apparatus that is itself the product of human labor. The objects of science are not dependent on human consciousness. And yet science happens in history, constrained by forms of social organization of a given type and of a given time. As such, existing social relations are a fetter upon science in its pursuit of the inhuman sensations of the nonhuman real.[38]

These prostheses of science—Wark follows Karen Barad and numerous others here in calling them 'apparatuses'—make available a radically *nonhuman* otherness.[39] Utilizing the word 'inhuman' in a very different way than Flusser did; *Molecular Red* draws a threefold distinction between the human, nonhuman, and inhuman.

As Slavoj Žižek notes in his review of this text: 'Crucial here is the distinction between nonhuman and inhuman: nonhuman resides at the same level as human; it is part of the ordinary world in which humans confront nonhuman things and processes. The apparatus is something different, neither human nor nonhuman but inhuman.'[40] Žižek further correctly notes:

> Although these apparatuses are made by humans and from part of our ordinary reality, they enable us [to] gain access to weird domains which are NOT part of our experiential human reality, from quantum oscillations to genomes...they enable us to discern the contours of a real that is not part of our reality. [Thus,] ...[t]he inhuman mediates the nonhuman to the human. This preserves the queer, *alien* quality of what can be produced by an apparatus—particle physics for example—without saying too much about the nonhuman in advance.'[41]

What is commendable about Wark's argument—and, indeed, a great deal of Žižek's thinking about science in general over his career—is the way in which it allows one to describe science and the Lacanian letter qua mathematical formula *in the Real* as profoundly *inhuman* prostheses that gives one access to the nonhuman Real.

This view of science and mathematics needs recourse to Lacan, largely because of how different it is from the perspective on science we have inherited from the phenomenological tradition. With Husserl, in particular, there has often been a rather steadfast argument that much of the human experiences of our 'life-world' really are not completely and totally 'alien' to the world(s) that are disclosed through science and all its prostheses, *pace* Žižek. As Pierre Kerszberg puts it in his 'Natural Science and the Experience of Nature,' for Husserlian phenomenology, '[t]he scientist is not a monstrous creature from outer space, but a human being equipped with a sense of being that belongs to us all, so that the concrete life-world in which we all live cannot but remain the "grounding soil" of the "true" world according to physics.'[42]

After the numerous ecological interventions from the new materialisms' camps, it seems that with twentieth-century science—from quantum mechanics to genetics and even environmental science that teaches one about objects that completely escape everyday existence—it gets harder and harder not to see this prioritizing of the human and even the *soil* as begging the question. Why is it not far more likely that science has so pulled away from this 'grounding soil' that to say otherwise is to privilege a human order of magnitude that need have no especial ontological privileging? Kerzsberg's essay—and phenomenology in general, one could argue—does grant that science has taught us to expand our understandings of the nonhuman world, that scientific knowledge shows that 'the electrons moving in highly elaborate circuits are just as "natural" as a table or a thunderstorm.'

Notwithstanding the fact that there are modes of being now that we access solely through abstractions (e.g., of mathematical formalism in the case of quantum mechanics), the phenomenologist can still wonder: '[D]espite those artifacts, and over and above them, isn't there some original nature that continues to provide a basis, a ground, a shelter'?[43] But, again, what if this wish for 'shelter' is yet another lure—just another way to be suspicious that the discoveries of science are not nearly as astonishing and narcissistically upsetting as they truly are—or, perhaps even worse, another way to still maintain humans as the 'monarchs of being'?[44] Flusser's demand that awareness of the degree to which scientific knowledge of orders of magnitude far outstretches the intuitions we have from the 'life-world' may indeed be just another way to domesticate and humanize the *radical otherness* that scientific knowledge unveils.

Kerzsberg argues that the scientist is no monstrous alien—perhaps not, but her knowledge certainly is. Ian Bogost, in thinking about the alien in general, says that the key question one must ask of the alien, of the radically foreign, is not '"Do you come in peace?" but rather, "What am I to you?"'[45] The natural sciences have given us the age of the Universe, and we know the Earth began the process of accretion billions of years ago. We know that life itself on this planet needed an inordinately ungraspable amount of time to get enough cyanobacteria cranking out oxygen to completely alter the entire planet's atmospheric composition, and science has taught us how old the genus *Homo* is.

Moreover, as Ray Brassier notes in his *Nihil Unbound*, the sciences also have told us a great deal about the future. For example, the Milky Way is on a crash-course trajectory with the Andromeda galaxy after another three billion years; the Sun will go red giant in four billion years; and somewhere around a trillion, trillion, trillion years from now, everything in the Universe will have been reduced back down into elementary particles.[46] Brassier is completely correct to say that '[p]hilosophers should be more astonished by such statements than they seem to be …' (Ibid., p. 50).

One could transfer Bogost's quip about aliens to this very (alien) knowledge: 'What am I to all this knowledge?' Perhaps the only legitimate answer is: 'Nothing at all.' These numbers stretch back to a point in time when there was no soil, no Earth to ground anything nor provide any 'shelter'; they also point to a future wherein '[t]he sun, our earth and your thought will have been no more than a spasmodic state of energy, an instant of established order, a smile on the surface of matter in a remote corner of the cosmos.'[47] Trying to deal with these drastic differences in scale granted by the natural sciences—trying to keep oneself solely within the Flusserian 'typical epistemology, ethics, and aesthetics' of a particular scale of reality—seems unthinkably difficult.

How do we get comfortable with the double-bind created by the fact that we know so many of these scales of magnitude 'overlap each other and interpenetrate' all while carving out a space of priority for 'the human scale'? What if they do not simply 'overlap and interpenetrate' each other, but create problematic contradictions between these scales? What if it is simply impossible to maintain the privileging of the human scale in all its humanist past within a world where 'we can no longer claim that our existence is special *as existence*,' as Bogost puts it?[48]

There is no doubt a great deal more to be said about Flusser's descriptions of our new reality *post*humanism, which is, in every way, a post-Galilean world. All the scales of magnitude seem to be fully continuous—they 'overlap each other and interpenetrate'—while at the same time being dotted with discontinuities and 'gray zones' where 'abysses gape.' When one looks at computer simulations of the evolution of the Universe, it becomes clear that there is just nothing smooth about it. Our Universe is indeed pockmarked with black holes, huge galaxies composed of incredibly massive systems that warp, contort, and distort the space around them in incredibly violent ways. Full of discontinuities, spaces in the Universe where, to be sure, 'abysses gape' as there are areas devoid of matter.

Žižek is fond of noting something analogous to this cosmological picture within the realm constrained by Darwinian Evolution. Any hint of a smooth, romantic view of the world is something we can no longer entertain: 'There is no Evolution: catastrophes and broken equilibriums are part of natural history; at numerous points in the past, life could have turned in an entirely different direction.'[49] The utter contingency of biological history goes just as well for cosmological history; both regimes, again, are shot through not with *meaning* but with abysses, discontinuities, 'catastrophes and broken equilibriums.' In other words, the aesthetics of the world, where different scales overlap and yet produce abysses, cannot be ordered toward the categories of harmony and balance.

Utilizing Lacanian categories to fundamentally upset these aesthetic ones so prided by Romantic conceptions of the nonhuman world makes psychoanalysis and ecological thinking into rather nice bedfellows. As a well-known anthology of ecological poetry recently noted, one of the key facets of this kind of poetry is how it so often formulates a critique of 'a form historically taken for granted—that of the singular, coherent self.'[50] The way in which the letter in the Real becomes a kind of 'excrement that has turned against its own progenitor' almost perfectly describes the traumatic impact of the mathematico–scientific apparatus's ability to access the nonhuman. Nobus already noted this trauma in his essay on the later Lacan work, which interprets this rupture as being one of the powers of the literary, that 'challenges the integrity of the Symbolic order.'[51]

This fundamental rupture seems to be another nice lens through which to read Ray Brassier's work (itself not an immediately fertile-looking ground for Lacanians, to be sure); he has been quite vocal in his argument that the very concepts of 'narrative' and 'meaning' have been thoroughly destabilized by the mathematical and theoretical sciences' use of the antisignifer of the letter. Narrative itself, far from providing some kind of great and comprehensive aesthetic whole, always has a hole in it somewhere, as Lacan knew so well.

In an interview with Marcin Rychter of *Kronos*, Brassier highlights the same history we have been discussing through Lacan's work:

> The emergence of modern mathematized natural science around the 16th [c]entury marks the point at which this way of making sense of ourselves and our world begins to unravel. …Over the course of a few centuries, the longstanding assumption that everything exists for a reason, that things are intrinsically purposeful and have been designed in accordance with a divine plan, is slowly but systematically dismantled. …Curved space-time, the periodic table, natural selection: *none of these are comprehensible in narrative terms.* Galaxies, molecules, and organisms are not *for* anything. Try as we might, it becomes increasingly difficult to construct a rationally plausible narrative about the world that satisfies our psychological need for stories that unfold from beginning, through crisis, to ultimate resolution.[52]

Brassier's argument, which again shows great similarity to Lacan's, that there is something strange that has happened with this rise of modern mathematized natural sciences—namely, that there has been a rupture between what he terms 'intelligibility' and 'meaning.' With post-Galilean science, 'conceptual rationality weans itself from the narrative structures that continue to prevail in theology and theologically inflected metaphysics.'

This occurrence, for Brassier—and for numerous others as well—'marks a decisive step forward in the slow process through which human rationality has gradually abandoned mythology, which is basically the interpretation of reality in narrative terms.' As he puts it, again holding nothing back: 'The world has no author and there is no story enciphered in the structure of reality. No narrative is unfolding in nature. …'[53] To argue otherwise is itself to try to thoroughly heal the wounding caused by scientific and mathematical knowledge itself—not to mention the ways in which this knowledge affects one's inability to (within the Lacanian register of the Imaginary) 'construct a rationally plausible narrative about the world that satisfies our psychological need for stories. …'

We are certainly creatures of the Imaginary and the Symbolic; however, at the same time, we are also creatures that are traversed and cut by apparatuses that touch the Real. This, of course, also means that we can come to some awareness of how some of our constructed stories attempt to avoid the traumatic nature of scientific knowledge's inhuman access to the nonhuman Real. Steven Shaviro is no doubt correct that ecological thinking requires us to 'stop telling ourselves the same old anthropocentric stories.'[54] Lacanian psychoanalysis cannot be easily included within such an anthology of nighttime stories. Lacan's thought is a kind of precondition not only for understanding the nightmares that plague everyone in the wake of these bedtime stories, but also a healthy antidote for hopefully grasping our current coordinates within the Anthropocene.

Notes

1. 'The Question Concerning Nature,' in *The Emerging Field of Environmental Hermeneutics*, ed. Forest Clingerman, et al. (New York: Fordham University Press, 2014), p. 224.
2. Ibid.
3. Adrian Johnston, *Prolegomena to Any Future Materialism, Volume 1: The Outcome of Contemporary French Philosophy* (Evanston: Northwestern University Press, 2013), p. 69.
4. Timothy Morton, *The Ecological Thought* (Cambridge: Harvard University Press, 2010), p. 32.

5. See Timothy Clark, *The Cambridge Introduction to Literature and the Environment* (New York: Cambridge University Press, 2011), for more on this splitting.
6. In *Writings*, ed. Andreas Ströhl (Minneapolis: University of Minnesota Press, 2002), p. 160.
7. Flusser (2002, p. 161).
8. Ibid.
9. Ibid., p. 164.
10. Ibid., pp. 163–164.
11. Carl Sagan, *Billions and Billions: Thoughts on Life and Death at the Brink of the Millennium* (New York: Ballantine, 1997), p. 11.
12. Flusser (2002), p. 161.
13. Jacques Lacan, 'Science and Truth,' in *Écrits: The First Complete Edition in English*, trans. Bruce Fink (New York: W.W. Norton, 2006), p. 728.
14. Hannah Arendt, *The Human Condition* (Chicago: University of Chicago Press, 1998), pp. 3, 4.
15. 'In 'Memory of Ernest Jones: On His Theory of Symbolism,' in *Écrits,* p. 596.
16. Jacques Lacan, *The Seminar of Jacques Lacan—Book XX: Encore On Feminine Sexuality, 1972–1973*, ed. J.-A. Miller, trans. Bruce Fink (New York: W. W. Norton, 1998), p. 43.
17. Jean-Claude Milner, 'The Doctrine of Science,' *Umbr(a): A Journal of the Unconscious, Science, and Truth* 1: 33–63, 50, 2000.
18. Tom Eyers, in *Cosmos and History: The Journal of Natural and Social Philosophy* 7(1): 155–166, 2011.
19. Ibid., p. 165.
20. Lacan, in *Ecrits*, trans. Bruce Funk (New York: W. W. Norton, 2006), p. 413.
21. Eyers (2011), p. 163.
22. Ibid., p. 162.
23. Dany Nobus, 'Illiterature,' in *Re-Inventing the Symptom: Essays on the Final Lacan* (New York: Other Press, 2002), pp. 19–43.
24. Ibid., p. 29.
25. Ibid.
26. Lacan, Seminar XIV: The Logic of Phantasy, January 18, 1967, trans. Cormac Gallagher, from unedited and unpublished French manuscripts. See also the session of May 10, 1967: 'There is only a single domain, it seems—and I am not sure about it—which has no relation with the

sexual act in so far as it concerns the truth; it is mathematics, at its point of confluence with logic. But I believe that this is what allowed Russell to say that one never knows whether what one is putting forward is true.'

27. See Karen Barad, *Meeting the Universe Halfway: Quantum Physics and the Entanglement of Matter and Meaning* (Durham: Duke University Press, 2007), p. 132: 'Language has been granted too much power.'
28. This is made most clear in Chapter 9 of Horowitz's *Divine Name Verification* (Brooklyn: Punctum Books, 2013), 'Philosophical Excursus: A Critique of "Object-Oriented Ontology,"' p. 98, especially.
29. Noah Horowitz, *Reality in the Name of God, or Divine Insistence: An Essay on Creation, Infinity, and the Ontological Implications of Kabbalah* (Brooklyn: Punctum Books, 2012).
30. Ibid., p. 89.
31. Ibid., p. 90. Weiss's article quoted by Horowitz is 'On the Matter of Language: The Creation of the World from Letters and Lacan's Perception of Letters as Real,' *The Journal of Jewish Thought and Philosophy* 17(1): 101–115, 2009.
32. Ibid.
33. Ibid.
34. Lacan (1998), p. 59. The previously cited session of Wednesday May 10, 1967 in Seminar XIV also supports this connection between mathematics, the (lack of) sexual relation, and the impossible.
35. Cary Wolfe, *What Is Posthumanism?* (Minneapolis: University of Minnesota Press, 2010), p xxvi.
36. Wolfe (2010), p. 6; emphasis mine.
37. See Wolfe's *Prolegomena to Any Future Materialism* for more on this critique.
38. Mackenzie Wark, *Molecular Red: Theory for the Anthropocene* (New York: Verso Books, 2015), p. 208.
39. Wark, 'The Capitolocene,' *Public Seminar*, October 15, 2015. http://www.publicseminar.org/2015/10/the-capitalocene/#.WAfPjKOZPBI. Accessed 14 Jun 2016.
40. Slavoj Žižek, 'Ecology Against Mother Nature. In Žižek on *Molecular Red.* http://www.versobooks.com/blogs/2007-ecology-against-mother-nature-slavoj-zizek-on-molecular-red. Accessed 26 May 2015.
41. Wark (2015a), p. 164.
42. Pierre Kerszberg, 'Natural Science and the Experience of Nature,' *Angelaki* 10(1): 189, 2005.

43. Ibid.
44. Levi Bryant, *The Democracy of Objects* (Ann Arbor: Open Humanities Press, 2011), p. 44.
45. Ian Bogost, *Alien Phenomenology, or What It's Like to Be a Thing* (Minneapolis: University of Minnesota Press, 2012), p. 133.
46. Ray Brassier, *Nihil Unbound: Enlightenment and Extinction* (New York: Palgrave Macmillan, 2007), pp. 49–50.
47. Jean-François Lyotard, *The Inhuman: Reflections on Time*, trans. Geoffrey Bennington and Rachel Bowlby (Stanford: Stanford University Press, 1993), pp. 11–12.
48. Bogost (2012), p. 8.
49. Slavoj Žižek, 'Nature and its Discontents,' *SubStance* 37(3): 56, 2008.
50. Ann Fisher-Wirth and Laura-Gray Street, *The Ecopoetry Anthology* (San Antonio: Trinity University Press, 2013), p. xxix.
51. Nobus (2002), p. 30.
52. Ray Brassier, 'I Am a Nihilist Because I Still Believe in Truth,' March 4, 2011. http://www.kronos.org.pl/index.php?23151,896. Accessed 14 Jul 2016; emphasis mine.
53. Ibid.
54. Quoted in Barad (2007), p. 132.

Bibliography

Arendt, Hannah. 1998. *The Human Condition*. Chicago: University of Chicago Press.

Barad, Karen. 2007. *Meeting the Universe Halfway: Quantum Physics and the Entanglement of Matter and Meaning*. Durham: Duke University Press.

Bogost, Ian. 2012. *Alien Phenomenology, or What It's Like to Be a Thing*. Minneapolis: University of Minnesota Press.

Brassier, Ray. 2007. *Nihil Unbound: Enlightenment and Extinction*. New York: Palgrave Macmillan.

———. 2011. I Am a Nihilist Because I Still Believe in Truth, March 4. http://www.kronos.org.pl/index.php?23151,896. Accessed 14 Jul 2016.

Bryant, Levi. 2011. *The Democracy of Objects*. Ann Arbor: Open Humanities Press.

Clark, Timothy. 2011. *The Cambridge Introduction to Literature and the Environment*. New York: Cambridge University Press.

Eyers, Tom. 2011. Lacanian Materialism and the Question of the Real. *Cosmos and History* 7 (1): 155–166.
Fisher-Wirth, Ann, and Laura-Gray Street. 2013. *The Ecopoetry Anthology*. San Antonio: Trinity University Press.
Flusser, Vilém. 2002. Orders of Magnitude and Humanism. In *Writings*, ed. Andreas Ströhl, 160–164. Minneapolis: University of Minnesota Press.
Horowitz, Noah. 2012. *Reality in the Name of God, or Divine Insistence: An Essay on Creation, Infinity, and the Ontological Implications of Kabbalah*. Brooklyn: Punctum Books.
———. 2013. *Divine Name Verification*. Brooklyn: Punctum Books.
Johnston, Adrian. 2013. *Prolegomena to Any Future Materialism, Volume 1: The Outcome of Contemporary French Philosophy*. Evanston: Northwestern University Press.
Kerszberg, Pierre. 2005. Natural Science and the Experience of Nature. *Angelaki* 10 (1): 187–199.
Lacan, Jacques. 1967. Seminar XIV: The Logic of Phantasy. Trans. Cormac Gallagher. From unedited and unpublished French manuscript.
———. 1998. *The Seminar of Jacques Lacan, Book XX: Encore On Feminine Sexuality, 1972–1973*. ed. J.-A. Miller and trans. Bruce Fink. New York: W. W. Norton.
———. 2006. *Écrits: The First Complete Edition in English*. Trans. Bruce Fink. New York: W. W. Norton.
Lyotard, Jean-Francois. 1993. *The Inhuman: Reflections on Time*. Trans. G. Bennington and R. Bowlby. Stanford: Stanford University Press.
McGrath, Sean. 2014. The Question Concerning Nature. In *The Emerging Field of Environmental Hermeneutics*, ed. Forest Clingerman et al. New York: Fordham University Press.
Milner, Jean-Claude. 2000. The Doctrine of Science. *Umbr(a): Science and Truth*, No. 1 (2000): 33–63.
Morton, Timothy. 2010. *The Ecological Thought*. Cambridge: Harvard University Press.
Nobus, Dany. 2002. Illiterature. In *Re-inventing the Symptom: Essays on the Final Lacan*, 19–43. New York: Other Press.
Sagan, Carl. 1997. *Billions and Billions: Thoughts on Life and Death at the Brink of the Millennium*. New York: Ballantine.
Wark, Mackenzie. 2015a. *Molecular Red: Theory for the Anthropocene*. New York: Verso Books.
———. 2015b. The Capitolocene. *Public Seminar*. http://www.publicseminar.org/2015/10/the-capitalocene/#.WAfPjKOZPBI. Accessed XX Mon 20XX.

Weiss, Tzahi. 2009. On the Matter of Language: The Creation of the World from Letters and Lacan's Perception of Letters as Real. *The Journal of Jewish Thought and Philosophy* 17 (1): 101–115.
Wolfe, Cary. 2010. *What Is Posthumanism?* Minneapolis: University of Minnesota Press.
Žižek, Slavoj. 2008. Nature and Its Discontents. *SubStance* 37 (3): 37–72.
———. 2015. Ecology Against Mother Nature. In Slavoj Žižek *Molecular Red.* New York: Verso Books. http://www.versobooks.com/blogs/2007-ecology-against-mother-nature-slavoj-zizek-on-molecular-red. Accessed XX Mon 20XX.

Lacanian Anti-Humanism and Freedom

Ed Pluth

There seem to be two basic ways of conceiving or modeling freedom in Lacan's work—an early one for which full speech is the primary concept or label, and a later one in which the psychoanalytic act plays this role. Although these two models bridge the gap between the early and the late Lacan, with all the differences that entails, they are closer to each other than one might suspect given all the other major theoretical shifts that occur. Both, at a minimum, can be considered exemplars of an antihumanist theory of freedom. This chapter considers only how the first concept, full speech, is antihumanist despite being couched in terms that suggest humanist assumptions.

But then again, does Lacan really have a theory of freedom at all? When Lacan was interviewed for Belgian television in 1972, the documentarian Françoise Wolff asked him: 'So, in a psychoanalysis, there is not a repression of freedom?'[1] Lacan laughed, and then added: 'Yes… these terms, the term, makes me laugh, yes. I never talk about freedom.'

E. Pluth (✉)
California State University, Chico, CA, USA

G. Basu Thakur, J.M. Dickstein (eds.), *Lacan and the Nonhuman*,
The Palgrave Lacan Series, DOI 10.1007/978-3-319-63817-1_6

Lacan was probably just trying to dismiss her concern about psychoanalysis and oppression by saying that he just never talks about freedom. But, of course, it is entirely false that Lacan never talked about freedom.

It is important, however, to consider this: When Lacan does talk about freedom, what is he actually doing? He is, in a sense, perhaps not really talking about it, because more often than not when he talks about freedom, he is critiquing a particular model of freedom—I'm calling it 'humanist' here, although labels (e.g., 'existentialist' and 'voluntarist)' would serve well too. His sustained critique of such freedom does not, perhaps, amount to really 'talking about' freedom in a positive fashion after all. Nonetheless, this will not do either; because even apart from his negative comments about freedom, Lacan in fact does talk more robustly about freedom than he led his interviewer to believe.

In Seminar II Lacan even went so far as to call psychoanalysis an 'apprenticeship in freedom.'[2] This is a delightfully paradoxical phrase: One has to be apprenticed into freedom, making it something far from a guaranteed existential condition of being human. This phrase expresses very quickly the strangeness of Lacan's (positive) antihumanist conception of freedom. Psychoanalysis is an apprenticeship in freedom; however, does this not taint the freedom acquired? (So, was not Wolff's, perhaps Foucauldian/Deleuzian, concern, right? Psychoanalysis is oppression masked as liberation? It makes one dependent on another for his or her very autonomy!) In a related claim from the same seminar, in what I take as another positive comment about freedom and psychoanalysis, evoking Mallarmé, Lacan said: 'The game is already played, the die already cast. It is already cast, with the following proviso, that we can pick it up again, and throw it anew.'[3] The psychoanalytic cure represents another throw of the die: change is present here, in some way.

But then is this change a free act? Is it the result of a free act? This is all still up in the air, and this is the point this chapter focuses on, about freedom in Lacanian theory: There is not only a critique of freedom in Lacan but also a rethinking of its parameters, such that freedom is not entirely off the map in Lacanian theory, and his discussions of it are not only and exclusively negative or critical. The trickier question is: How is it conceived positively? What follows discusses how Lacan's thoughts about machines in the second seminar can be used to sketch out how this positive theory might look; and they also will show how the concept of 'full speech,' used at the time as a key concept in the psychoanalytic cure, which is used as a term for the free 'act' here, is not as humanist as it sounds.

Machines, Animals, and Freedom

One should give Lacan a lot of credit for posing as a Heidegger-enthusiast in the 1950s while at the same time pursuing and embracing technological and machinic conceptions of the human. Heidegger's technophobia is well known, while Lacan's discussions of machines, codes, and cybernetic systems are in fact the best places to look for the positive outlines of his antihumanist theory of freedom.

Why did Lacan think that a study of machines, codes, and cybernetic systems would tell us something about human freedom, rather than telling us what would be the more obvious, expected thing: That we are programmed, that the die is already cast, and that we are simply repeating ourselves without knowing what the plan is? Consider Lacan's frequent comparisons of the unconscious to an old tickertape machine, cranking out associations and chains of Signifiers. Is this not a comparison that renders us more determined than we ever thought? In addition, we could take as the very image of *homo-Freudians* the poor individual Lacan likes to refer to with a 'codicil' tattooed on her skull—the idea is that she is walking around bearing a message, tattooed on her from birth, of which she is entirely ignorant; however, this message is her essence because it determines her.

Despite all this, there is a surprising turn of events in Lacan's discussion of machines in Seminar II. Machines, he says, are freer than animals. Consider this key passage from Lacan's second seminar:

> The philosophical criticisms made of strictly mechanistic research assume the machine to be deprived of freedom. It would be very easy to prove to you that the machine is much freer than the animal.

Already Lacan is saying that when one is studying structures and the power of the Symbolic (in a sense the whole orientation of Seminar II), it might look like one is studying a variety of determinism; however, this is not the case at all! He continues: 'The animal is a jammed machine. It's a machine with certain parameters that are no longer capable of variation.'

It is not the case, then, that there are machines on the one hand and animals, nonmachines, on the other. Lacan is suggesting here that it is machines all the way through, so to speak: Animals are simply on one end of a machine-spectrum. Besides, they are jammed machines. This suggests that the principles governing machines, by contrast, can vary. Certain types of codes and structures are, unexpectedly perhaps, precisely what allow for variation. So, not being sufficiently subjected to a certain type of code would limit one's capacity for variation, which must be a synonym for freedom:

> 'And why? Because the external environment determines the animal, and turns it into a fixed type.'

It is exclusively about animals that Lacan elects to refer to determination; that is, when he is talking about an 'external environment'—an environment external to a structure, a code—that limits what the code can do. Thus, animals are determined because of the lack of code-variation and because of their fixed relationship to their external environments. In one respect, Lacan could be said to be following a Heideggerian line of thinking here. In other words, vegetables and minerals would have no world (they would not be machines at all), animals have a world but are world-impoverished (i.e., *weltarm*) because they are transfixed, or fully absorbed, in their worlds (i.e., jammed machines).

The next, rather un-Heideggerian, step would be to say that Dasein, however, *has* a world (because they are closer to 'pure machines'). Here is what Lacan says:

> 'It is in as much as, compared to the animal, we are machines, that is to say something decomposed [décomposé], that we possess greater freedom.'[4]

'Decomposed' is perhaps not the best translation of the French *décomposé* but it can suggest the right associations—not something that decays so much as something that can be broken down into parts, but also analyzed bit by bit. What is it about machines, and their being able to be broken down and analyzed, that affords them greater freedom?

The analogy Lacan is working on here seems simple: machines are to animals as language is to instinct. Animals thus are fixed and jammed because of the limits of their languages. But there is something funny about this rather straightforward analogy, something missing from it, that becomes clearer later. Although machines are used to illustrate the height of language's presence and functioning, of its effects, the significant point Lacan is making in this seminar about machines (and this contrasts with us, most of the time), turns out to be that their superior freedom is because they do not interpret, as *we* (now more like the jammed machines than animals are) do when it comes to using language. The connection between machines and languages is a connection that actually gets rid of what seems to be so important about language from our normal perspective—its capacity for meaning, which the unconscious-machine will do without.

This is exemplified in Lacan's discussion of games. The fact that machines could outperform people at a game (e.g., odds and evens) was a huge deal for Lacan at the time—perhaps not such a surprise for us who are beaten by computers at all sorts of things regularly. The game of odds and evens that Lacan had his public play during that seminar was supposed to be an illustration of how difficult it is for us to be and to act, and to think, in a truly random manner; despite ourselves, we look for patterns because we cannot help but guess at meanings and intentions. (Consider the well-known fact that a series of 'random numbers' generated by a human being almost never contains any repetition: the absence of such repetition is a good indication that the sequence was generated by a human. Our understanding or our beliefs about what randomness 'looks like' corrupts our ability to generate a random sequence.)

To be conscious is, to paraphrase Sartre, to be condemned to meaning and interpretation. In this respect, we would indeed seem to be closer to the 'jammed machines' than animals are (if not worse, because of our lack of any smooth fit with our environment); we stupidly insist on a return to the familiar. We always are looking for the same thing, for the pattern we already know, or believe should exist. We are caught up in mimesis.

Think of the mirroring method referred to by Dupin in Poe's 'Purloined Letter,' a method Lacan ridicules in Seminar II as well as in the *Écrits*—the young man who was a champion at odds and evens would succeed by imitating the facial expressions of his opponents.[5] Once he got the facial expression right, his opponent's way of thinking would come to him, and he would be able to divine what his opponent would do next and win. If only it were so easy.

Lacan is claiming that machines possess a freedom superior to that of animals (and to us, for the most part) precisely because they do not fall for the lures of imitation and are therefore capable of a truer spontaneity or 'variation.' In other words, machines are more purely creatures of the Symbolic, and are freed from the Imaginary; they do not try to guess intent and hidden meaning—in short, they do not interpret. For this reason they are more 'free,' where this means now something like 'truly autonomous' and free from repetitive pattern-seeking and meaning-seeking.

Freedom in Full Speech

Although an animal is subject to a code, something like a machine then, it is still immersed in its environment, dependent on its external world. Yet it is a machine's total immersion in its code that ironically gives it more freedom—on the assumption that the code itself contains the capacity for variation. The surprising result of Lacan's thinking in Seminar II is that the place in human practice in which we would find the same kind of 'greater freedom' found in machines is right where it would not seem to be at all. That is, in Lacan's otherwise very humanist-sounding idea of full speech, provided this is seen as a manifestation of the unconscious.

Why call this antihumanist? Because we are jammed machines when we interpret, when we look for meaning, when we are sensitive to the enigmas of human speech; it is precisely there where we appear to be most human—open to the other, open to ambiguity, considerate, charitable, self-doubting. Also, by contrast, it is when the machine of language is instead left to go on autopilot, as it were, that a greater (Symbolic, or 'of the symbolic'?) freedom emerges. I argue here that this is what full speech actually is about.

Full speech is such a problematic concept in Lacan's work, one hardly commented on any more, perhaps because of its very title and its inevitable opposition to empty speech—an opposition that can take us in so many wrong directions. To rehabilitate the concept of full speech, what we would have to do is portray empty speech as something that is in fact expressively full; it is the very kind of speech in which we are in fact trying to communicate at all, authentically or inauthentically. No matter in what mode we are trying to express ourselves and, reciprocally, trying to figure out our own and the other's meanings—all of this is the speech of the 'jammed machines' or the animals that we otherwise are.

Readers of Lacan who know their Heidegger, such as Muller and Richardson, described empty speech in the following terms: It was when 'the subject speaks of himself as if he were an other, as if his own ego were alienated from the deeper subjectivity that properly assumes "his desire".' [6] This reference to a 'deeper subjectivity' about which one should be speaking makes it sound as if full speech would resemble Heideggerian authenticity, and that it would entail a mode of speaking in which one truly says what one is. The danger in understanding both full speech and empty speech this way (i.e., in expressivist terms) is that it sounds like it is possible to avoid empty speech by just speaking about oneself truthfully and honestly, perhaps in a confrontation with one's real self, or one's real need.

Nevertheless, the point is that nothing would be emptier either, from Lacan's perspective, insofar as such speech is still communicative, expressive, and—the main problem, perhaps—meaningful at all. Thus, what is being suggested here is that Lacanian full speech, as a manifestation of the unconscious, is in some way noncommunicative, nonexpressive, and more properly aligned with nonsense. This is how we should interpret the discussion of machines, languages/codes, and freedom in Seminar II.

Inspired by that discussion, full speech should be thought of instead as an almost automatic, machinic, flat, nonsensical speech act. These might strike one as descriptors of empty speech—which seems like it should be a meaningless blah blah blah. But then again, this is only if we let the phrase 'empty speech' evoke, erroneously, Heidegger's notion from *Being and Time* of *Gerede* (idle talk), about which Heidegger wrote that 'when Da-sein maintains itself in idle talk, it is—as being-in-the-world—cut off from the primary and primordially genuine relations of being toward the world, toward *Mitda-sein*, toward being-in itself.'[7] In addition, 'all genuine understanding, interpreting, and communication, rediscovery and new appropriation come about in it [idle talk] and out of it and against it.'[8]

Heidegger here opposes a superficial, everyday understanding and interpretation to a more genuine one; however, this more genuine and authentic speech is just a more genuine form of 'understanding, interpreting, and communication'—it is still on the same scale as they are. This is not the way to understand the opposition, in Lacan, between empty speech and full speech because in full speech, communication and expression, I argue, are not really involved.

Heidegger's opposition of genuine understanding to idle talk conforms to an expressivist model. Even some of Lacan's standard examples of full speech, such as 'you are my wife' or 'you are my master,' suggest this. Yet these standard Lacanian examples can be preserved as models of full (nonexpressive) speech if we think of them as things said that reveal the speaker has a commitment he did not know he had; that is, if we think of them as moments in which the speaker says something she did not know she meant, saying more than she wanted to say. Is this to say that full speech is performative: That it makes what it says? Can it be both performative and nonexpressive?

The reason why it would not qualify as performative, at least not in Austin's sense, is that Lacanian full speech does not consist of an addition of conscious assent to what is being said—'I say this now and I know I am saying it and I really mean it and fully commit myself to it.' The absence of this knowledge would make a speech act infelicitous. Yet full speech is precisely this; it reveals something *to which I have already assented*. It shows me where I was, so to speak, without knowing I was there; and the subject's surprise at such an utterance, as well as its resistance, needs to be highlighted here. Such surprise and resistance is what is involved in any manifestation of the unconscious, after all.

By contrast, empty speech would involve statements that can always be doubted, statements that may or may not reveal something about oneself as elusive, as well as indifferent statements that one can take or leave; statements that are, then, primarily directed toward an Other to get one recognized, to get demands recognized, and so on. In full speech, 'I' am speaking the commitment, the attachment, or however you want to characterize it; nevertheless, I am also surprised not only by what I say but also by the fact that what I say 'speaks my being,' *as* it were, more truly than I wish, such that it is impossible (empty?) to take it back or modify it.

What does this take on full speech have to do with freedom and machines? Again, what needs to be emphasized about full speech is its antihumanism—how it does not fit into the humanist expressive paradigm and the notion of the full presence to oneself. The humanist subject is surprised and bothered by what happens in a moment of full speech (one could say that it produces only the 'split' subject); one would have to imagine full speech as something like the voice of the Other emerging from oneself in a pure form—a voice that is Other but of course 'more you than you.' So, it is entirely too vague to explain full speech in terms of a speech that 'aims at truth,' even though Lacan himself said something like this in Seminar I, where he also said that it performs.[9]

In addition, in his response to Hyppolite's piece in the *Écrits*, Lacan wrote that 'full speech is defined by the fact that it is identical to what it speaks about.'[10] This is a strange and difficult idea. I am arguing that full speech is not about communication, expression, or meaning but rather it is a sort of 'revelation'—a term Lacan uses a few times in the context of explaining full speech. For example, 'the Freudian novelty compared to St. Augustine is the revelation…of these subjective "lived points" at which a speech emerges that surpasses the discoursing subject.'[11] This is exactly what full speech is; yet these moments of revelation have the status of nonsensical utterances as far as the expressing subject is concerned. They take that subject by surprise.

Madrun Sarup claimed:

> Lacan sees speech that carries the illusion of the intact ego as empty, in the Imaginary register: the subject does not speak but is spoken. Full speech follows the acceptance of the self as existing in the domain of inter-subjectivity; one ceases to speak of oneself as an object. […T]o attain full speech means to cease to speak of oneself as an object.[12]

Nevertheless, speaking, or producing, oneself as an object is, I say, pretty much what happens in full speech. In full speech, the subject is 'spoken' as well or 'gets itself spoken' even more so than in empty speech. In full speech, it is an 'Other discourse' that speaks; therefore full speech is more like a formation of the unconscious, more like a slip of the tongue or a parapraxis, than a moment of authenticity and fully self-conscious resoluteness.

Despite Lacan's discourse about psychoanalysis at this time as a 'reconciliation' with the 'it thinks' (*Wo Es war…soll Ich warden*), there is something about the moment of freedom in full speech that we can never become one with because what it presents, and produces, is exactly the divided subject. Perhaps the entire difficulty with the topic of freedom in Lacanian theory can be found in the fact that he thinks of the freedom of a subject divided from itself, and with itself. So, what if the 'apprenticeship in freedom' that psychoanalysis is supposed to be involves a rewrite of Freud's famous claim about morality, only this time in terms of freedom. Where Freud said that we are more moral than we think and less moral than we believe, Lacan is saying that we are both more and less free than we think.

Žižek wrote, in one of his most famous quotes, that, precisely because we 'feel free,' it is difficult to think about our un-freedom; and thinking this defacto un-freedom is an important task for ideology critique.[13] Perhaps this task can be accompanied by an attempt to think about a freedom, which, I emphasize, also may be said to happen at times, but in a mode we are not keen to recognize, and that may not at all make us 'feel free' because it is in a more machinic mode. This would be what an anti-humanist theory of freedom does for everyone.

Postscript

This is admittedly a strange way to think about freedom: It is nonconscious, it is nonexpressive, it has nothing to do with the will, or with self-actualization. To conclude, I want to consider a quote from an interview Peter Hallward did with Alain Badiou:

> Lin Piao—someone rarely mentioned these days—once said, at the height of the Cultural Revolution, that the essential thing was to be, at a revolutionary conjunction, both its actor and its target. I quite like this formula.

> Yes, we are actors, but in such a way that we are targeted by, carried away by, and struck by the event.[14]

If full speech can serve as a model of (positive) freedom in Lacanian theory, one of its important features appears to be its double nature—agency on one level and passivity on another. This chapter has been claiming, basically, that in full speech the humanist subject is overwhelmed by and spoken by some other agency. The idea that one is both agent and target in full speech, however, seems appropriate, though it is not without problems, which have been touched on briefly. How should one think about this 'other agency'?

Probably no one did more to problematize the entire notion of agency in the Western philosophical tradition than Heidegger, a point that is brought out well in Reiner Schürmann's study in *Heidegger on Being and Acting: From Principles to Anarchy*. For him 'anarchy'—acting without purpose, being without purpose, the absence of a governing principle—is found in what he takes to be the ultimate Heideggerian ethic. *Gelassenheit*: the idea that one must do what presence does. 'Anarchy' means just this for Schürmann—doing what presence does.

One way to think of this, Schürmann says, is to put it alongside the Christian mystic Meister Eckhart's famous injunction to live a life without 'why':

> [A]fter one of the more direct developments of what one could call ontological anarchy—expressed, as it happens, by the concept of 'life without why,' attributed to Master Eckhart (via Angelus Silesius)—Heidegger concludes: 'At the deepest base of his being, man only truly is when, in his own manner, he is like the rose—without why.'[15]

That this 'anarchy'—being and acting 'without why'—is supposed to serve as a version of antihumanist freedom in Heidegger is clear when Schürmann points out its opposition to key conceptions of freedom from figures in the philosophical, humanist tradition, as follows:

> To say that at the age of closure acting becomes free, this means, of course, that it liberates itself from 'principles.' [...] *Being free is doing what presence does*: letting all things be. Freedom is discovered then as the letting-be of

> being, as entry into an aletheo-logical constellation. This freedom no longer has anything to do with Aristotelian deliberative choice, the Augustinian 'will divided against itself,' Kantian causality and 'moral auto-determination' or even the 'fundamental choice in which I decide my own being' of Sartre. All these concepts situate freedom, if not in a faculty of the mind, at least in man.[16]

Nonetheless, even in this Heideggerian antihumanist version of freedom, agency is not entirely eluded; it is simply placed beyond humanity, and in what being does. Freedom, for us, consists of letting this happen.

Although critical of a tradition that locates agency in the individual, whether in consciousness or the will, Schürmann shows that Heidegger does not develop a concept of freedom that dispenses with agency altogether. This is probably not possible: without agency, the word 'freedom' just does not work. What Lacan is doing with both freedom and agency, however, topologically, is of greater interest, I contend, than Heidegger's decentering move. Rather than simply decentering agency (i.e., putting it in another location), Lacan, dialectically, splits the concept in two—in freedom, we are both agents and targets. Any theory of self-actualization might be understood to be saying the same thing; that is, we realize and actualize what we are. Lacan's is not a theory of self-actualization, however. The split subject does not allow for such a reading.

Why not? Lacan struggles with this issue in 'The Instance of the Letter.' I have in mind the passage in which he wonders whether the unconscious is just some Other agency that is really in charge of us, instead of consciousness. Lacan rejected this view when he wrote:

> Is what thinks in my place, then, another ego? Does Freud's discovery represent the confirmation, at the level of psychological experience, of Manichaeism? There can, in fact, be no confusion on this point: what Freud's research introduced us to was not some more or less curious cases of dual personality.[17]

So no, there are not two agents. What Lacan rejects here, however, is only the view that the unconscious is another Ego, or a more genuine Ego, that is actually in charge. Later, Lacan claims that what he wants to do is preserve the 'radical heteronomy that Freud's discovery shows gaping within man.'[18] Rather than dual agency, this should be thought of as a split agency, of the kind seen in full speech, in which the source appears at first to be other than the target, but the target is led to change itself and recognize itself in the foreign-seeming source. A more Hegelian than Heideggerian story, of course.

The topic of Heideggerian 'letting being be' is brought up here because it seems that one can take it, as Schürmann does, to involve a radical version of some kind of ontological freedom. Heidegger is getting at a kind of freedom that lies behind certain ways of thinking, maybe certain ways of acting. But to say that in something like full speech we are both its actor and its target is to suggest something else. For one thing, full speech is nothing like a persistent ontological background, something always already going on, behind whatever other kinds of speaking happen; instead it is a momentary, transitory, more event-like thing.

Notes

1. Jacques Lacan, 'Conference de Louvain Suivie d'un Entretien avec Françoise Wolff,' 1972, Videotape.
2. Lacan, *The Seminar of Jacques Lacan, Book II: The Ego in Freud's Theory and in the Technique of Psychoanalysis, 1954–1955.*, ed. Jacques-Alain Miller, trans. Sylvana Tomaselli (New York: W. W. Norton, 1991), p. 108.
3. Ibid, p. 219.
4. Ibid., p. 31.
5. Lacan, in *Ecrits* (2006), p. 14.
6. John P. Muller and William J. Richardson, *Lacan and Language: A Reader's Guide to Ecrits* (Madison: International Universities Press, 1994), p. 70.
7. Martin Heidegger, *Being and Time*, trans. Joan Stambaugh (Albany: SUNY Press, 1996), p. 159.
8. Ibid.
9. Lacan, *The Seminar of Jacques Lacan, Book I: Freud's Papers on Technique, 1953–1954*, trans. John Forrester (New York: W. W. Norton, 1991), p. 188.
10. Lacan (2006), p. 319.
11. Ibid., p. 407.

12. Madrun Sarup, *Jacques Lacan* (Toronto: University of Toronto Press, 1992), p. 55.
13. Slavoj Žižek, *Welcome to the Desert of the Real: Five Essays on September 11th and Related Dates*, (London: Verso, 2002), p. 2.
14. Alain Badiou, *Ethics: An Essay on the Understanding of Evil*, trans. Peter Hallward (London: Verso, 2001), p. 125.
15. Rainer Schürmann, *Heidegger on Being and Acting: From Principles to Anarchy* (Bloomington: Indiana University Press, 1987), p. 19.
16. Ibid., p. 109; emphasis added.
17. Lacan (2006), p. 435.
18. Ibid., p. 436.

Bibliography

Badiou, Alain. 2001. *Ethics: An Essay on the Understanding of Evil.* Trans. Peter Hallward. London: Verso.

Heidegger, Martin. 1996. *Being and Time.* Trans. Joan Stambaugh. Albany: SUNY Press.

Lacan, Jacques. 1972. Jacques Lacan. Conférence de Louvain Suivie d'un Entretien avec Francoise Wolff. Videotape.

———. 1991. *The Seminar of Jacques Lacan, Book Two: The Ego in Freud's Theory and in the Technique of Psychoanalysis, 1954–1955*. Ed. Jacques-Alain Miller. Trans. Sylvana Tomaselli. New York: W. W. Norton.

———. 2006. *Écrits: The First Complete Edition in English.* Trans. Bruce Fink. New York: W. W. Norton.

Muller, John P., and William J. Richardson. 1994. *Lacan and Language: A Reader's Guide to Ecrits*. Madison: International Universities Press.

Sarup, Madrun. 1992. *Jacques Lacan*. Toronto: University of Toronto Press.

Schürmann, Rainer. 1987. *Heidegger on Being and Acting: From Principles to Anarchy*. Bloomington: Indiana University Press.

Zizek, Slavoj. 2002. *Welcome to the Desert of the Real: Five Essays on September 11th and Related Dates*. London: Verso.

The Sovereign Signifier: Agamben and the Nonhuman

Paul Eisenstein

Giorgio Agamben's invocations of Sovereignty and Law would appear, on their face, to vex his relationship to a Lacanian conception of the nonhuman. At the heart of this vexed relationship is the seeming fealty Agamben's analyses pay to Michel Foucault. In the Introduction to his *Homo Sacer: Sovereign Power and Bare Life*, Agamben writes that in his final years, Foucault had appeared to orient his analysis of Power according to 'two distinct directives for research':

> [O]n the one hand, the study of the *political techniques* (such as the science of the police) with which the State assumes and integrates the care of the natural life of individuals into its very center; on the other, the examination of the *technologies of the self* by which processes of subjectivization bring the individual to bind himself to his own identity and consciousness and, at the same time, to an external power.[1]

To anyone familiar with Foucault's work, these two directives are hardly surprising. Agamben, for his part, appears to accept the basic two-pronged

P. Eisenstein (✉)
Otterbein University, Westerville, OH, USA

G. Basu Thakur, J.M. Dickstein (eds.), *Lacan and the Nonhuman*,
The Palgrave Lacan Series, DOI 10.1007/978-3-319-63817-1_7

thesis when it comes to analyzing Power, which is to say that he sees how the workings of disciplinary power are inseparable from processes that belong to the very advent of subjectivity, and the entire attachment or reduction of the body and its sensations to something called an Individual Subject.[2]

To the extent that Agamben has a quarrel with Foucault, it is that the latter never names or locates the exact point of intersection in the body of Power itself 'at which techniques of individualization and totalizing procedures converge.'[3] He likens this place of meeting to 'a vanishing point that the different perspectival lines of Foucault's inquiry (and, more generally, of the entire Western reflection on power) converge toward without reaching.'[4] It is the self-proclaimed achievement of Agamben's work to have reached and rendered visible this vanishing point in the figure of the *homo sacer*—the casualty of a sovereign, legal decision, the life that is included in a political order 'solely in the form of its exclusion.'[5] This 'obscure figure of archaic Roman law' offers, according to Agamben, nothing less than 'the key by which not only the sacred texts of sovereignty but also the very codes of political power will unveil their mysteries.'[6]

How, and in what way, does the figure of the *homo sacer* render visible the mystery of political Power? The answers provided by Agamben to this question are, in a significant way, historicist: Western politics gets founded on the exclusion of an exemplar of biological life (the *homo sacer*)—on a sovereign decree that divides human and nonhuman life, privileging the former and permitting violence against the latter. The *homo sacer* is precisely the person who can be killed without it being considered a crime.[7]

In modernity, this fracturing decree takes on a paradoxically doleful hue. In antiquity, the *homo sacer* is distinguished from the rights-bearing citizen, relegated to and associated with a form of living that is the abject, sacred, denuded substance of life itself; in modernity, however, the beneficiaries of the fracturing decree want that sacredness for their own lives and societies as well. Thus, for Agamben, this fracturing decree comes to bewitch modern democracies, the citizens of which come to imagine a freedom and plenitude in bare life itself, in the organic life of their community, if only it could be rid of its (ostensible) contaminants.

Agamben follows Foucault's theorization of the emergence of 'biopower' here because it is Foucault who first isolates the way in which biological life itself becomes a matter of political concern. For Foucault, biological life and its survival was once not something that concerned politics. Indeed, what Foucault calls 'the fact of living' was a concern that appeared only episodically (and apolitically) amid death-producing events (e.g., epidemics and famine), events that were understood to fall fundamentally outside of human control. As control over the conditions of existence grew during the eighteenth century—largely because of improved agricultural techniques and also of the rise of scientific disciplines that constructed, or even invented, life[8]—an opportunity emerged for human subjects to understand themselves as the bearers of life in a living world that could be known and transformed.

The double-valenced opportunity Foucault describes amounts to this: It is only life's *respite from* the vicissitudes of death that enables its capture by biopower, enables it to pass 'into knowledge's field of control and power's sphere of intervention.'[9] Life becomes the province of the State, which has an interest now in the living bodies of its citizens. A vast array of disciplines and institutions are developed that produce, articulate, disseminate, and ultimately regulate the truth of life. (Psychoanalysis and the psychoanalytic session would be seen to be part of this production/regulation.) The concept and exercise of Truth itself, as Foucault would put it, 'lays down the law.'[10] Biological life and its putative enjoyment become the object of political strategies and struggles—the thing of unsurpassed value when it comes to politics today.

What unites and explains phenomena as otherwise disparate as Nazism, the spectacle-ridden society of late capitalist consumerism, and the War on Terror is thus the increased politicization of biological life—the attempt to secure and enjoy natural life directly or immediately. The fantasmatic, besieged pleasures of biological existence therefore lie at the source of the horrible violence of the twentieth and twenty-first centuries, which at times leads Agamben to follow Foucault in calling for a new way of conceiving politics altogether—a politics, he says, 'no longer founded on the *exceptio* of bare life.'[11] Only an entirely new way of thinking about politics can free one from the way sovereign decisions politicize biological life via acts of Law that include life in and through the act of excluding it.

This relationship of 'inclusive exclusion' is, for Agamben, 'the originary form of law.'[12] From this Foucauldian standpoint, it would appear that there is no way of redeeming Law, or making it somehow fairer or just. It is not a question of looking to and overseeing more just incarnations of the Lacanian Law, the essence of which is 'to divide up, distribute, or reattribute everything that counts as *jouissance*.'[13] Political struggle is not a question of shoring up the Law against its manipulability, of fighting for better or more equitable distributions of jouissance, of relocating the source of the Law's emergence in the people as opposed to the Sovereign. The implications of the trenchant observations in a book such as Richard Rubenstein's *The Cunning of History*—that 'the Nazis committed no crime at Auschwitz,' that 'no laws were broken and no crimes committed at Auschwitz,' that the 'Jews were executed in accordance with German Law'—are those of someone who believes in the liberal–democratic version of Law and in the capacity of a *polis* to check the Sovereign's manipulation of it.[14]

On this view, only better and fairer laws, laws that respect the rights and dignity of all people, can create something like a more just and humane society. For Foucault, however, the problem is that Law *touches or appropriates the human and questions of pleasure at all*. In a clear evocation of Foucault, and in a way seemingly at odds with psychoanalysis, Agamben calls for a politics 'beyond every idea of' or in 'relation to' Law.[15] This kind of politics stands to change—in the direction of nonappropriation and nondomination—the very way we encounter living and inanimate beings.[16] Collapsing the human–nonhuman distinction frees in a radical way both parties from the inclusion–exclusion problematic. The nonhuman escapes the violence visited on it by the human, while human subjects themselves are afforded the putatively liberating chance—to invoke the name of Gerard Bruns's book—to 'cease to be human.'[17]

Which Bare Life?

When Agamben calls for a politics no longer founded on the Law-executing *exceptio* of bare life, we should, however, ask: Which bare life is he talking about? This question is pertinent because it seems to me that there are two bare lives in Agamben's analysis of the exception/exclusions created by Law. By this, I mean that there are two distinct sovereignties in Agamben's work.

The first is a sovereignty that happens historically, that exercises its powers in ways that marginalize other living creatures. This is a sovereignty that *need not have* exercised its Power in the way that it does. The designation of prisoners in the so-called War on Terror as 'enemy combatants'—and their indefinite detention at Guantánamo, without ever being accused of a crime—is one example of this exercise of Sovereignty. The second, however, is one that is constitutive—a sovereignty the exercise of which, insofar as we live in a properly social world, already has happened. This is a sovereignty that is logically necessary. If the first Sovereignty is exemplified by actual victims of political violence (e.g., the refugee or immigrant, the African-American victim of police violence, the disposable worker), the second has no actuality and no exemplar.

This second sovereignty produces a nonhuman form of life that is necessarily and entirely *conceptual*, the result of a different sort of Sovereign decision, one having to do with the law-bearing function of language itself. In his lone reference to Hegel in *Homo Sacer*, Agamben suggests that we have Hegel to thank for letting one see how the primordial Sovereign is language itself, because it is only with the advent of language that the illusion of something meaningful prior to language appears. We experience this advent as undoing the tie to natural biological life but in truth there was no prior tie, no subjective experience of it. The logical necessity of this dynamic, Agamben writes, makes plain 'the bond of inclusive exclusion to which a thing is subject because of the fact of being in language, of being named. To speak is, in this sense, always to "speak the law".'[18]

The notion that an individual speaking speaks the Law or expresses the bond of inclusive–exclusion has its antecedent in Hegel's critique of sense-certainty in *The Phenomenology*; this book definitively establishes the extent to which the immediacy of anything captured by language is always already (and necessarily) a vanished immediacy. As Hegel illustrates it, actual, discrete particulars '*cannot be reached* by language': The instant someone names or describes a particular thing (e.g., 'this bit of paper'), the absolute particularity of this thing has been replaced by the words used to refer to or describe it.[19] One cannot 'say' a particular thing without the sound of the saying itself becoming a particular thing, forsaking its referential function—its ability to enable one to *think* the particular thing being designated or to grasp how there are many actual, discrete particulars.

The phrase 'this bit of paper,' after all, can refer to many different bits of paper. For Hegel, then, the cognizance or retention of particularity is paradoxically inseparable from its sacrifice. The valorized sensuousness of the particulars of sensory perception is always a retroactive construction, an effect of a nomenclatural foreclosure, which means that whatever we are able to designate meaningfully about such details is already the result of our having 'spoken the law.'

Hegel applies this thesis regarding the fantasy of sense-certainty explicitly to biological life itself (what he calls 'mere' life) in part three of the greater *Logic*, where he makes plain the extent to which any and all invocations of mere life must reckon with the way such life gets cognized. Indeed, in the final section of his book, Hegel traces the way cognition itself forges and maintains an identity between its own idea of natural life and natural life itself *even as* it announces their diremption. As Hegel sees it, philosophy goes farther than sciences (e.g., physics or psychology) because these sciences are content to generate or determine general laws based on empirical considerations. Philosophy, however, grasps the way the Absolute Idea or Absolute Notion clarifies the way the very appearance of empirical entities that are different from thinking is, at the same time, unifying.

To recognize this is to have arrived at the Absolute Idea or Absolute Notion—the thought of thought that overcomes all opposition. Hegel's *Science of Logic* is a unique science for this reason because it does not separate form and content. Thinking is not the mere form of cognition, as if content (or matter) came from somewhere else. Thinking is not, in other words, some sort of empty, external vessel that arrives at real or concrete material in order to fill itself up and become genuine knowing. On the contrary, as Hegel insists (crediting Plato and the Ancients): '[T]the knowledge of things obtained through thinking is alone what is true in them, that is, things not in their immediacy but as first raised into the form of thought, as things *thought*.'[20] What Hegel calls the 'most important proposition of philosophy' is precisely the *ideality* of all finite entities or things.[21]

These Hegelian propositions here do necessarily entail hierarchy. Human cognition, for Hegel, *is* inescapably a higher stage than life, and the subject who can cognize the very terms of cognition itself vis-à-vis the natural or animal world *is* in fact the fulcrum of an egalitarian politics. The insights into animal or biological life that thinks such insights *as thought*—as determinations that are *the essential nature of* or an expression of logical kinship between thinking and objects—are truer than insights into, or practices of, animal or biological life that claim to have evaded thinking, or that emanate directly from everything that thinking is said to negate (e.g., the body, one's animal urges, mere life, etc.). This is what Hegel means when he insists that the '[i]dea of life…remain enclosed within the form of the Notion' and should not take its cue from actual forms of natural life itself.[22]

When we consider the conceptual or logical conditions that undergird our very cognizance of biological life, we can see that there is no getting intelligibly to the thing itself. The very words 'biological' or 'natural life' are, before they are anything else, abstract—an idea. Biological or natural life, in other words, has no intelligible meaning outside of, or prior to, the signifying act that conditions its emergence, and it is this signifying act that always already signals a primordial alienation from nature. Catherine Malabou beautifully distills the contours of this alienation when she invokes 'signification's impossible state of nature.'[23] The politics that aims to reconcile signification and nature is one that ignores its own constitutive conditions.

In naming language as Sovereign, Agamben enables one to conclude that there is a sovereignty that is logical or Notional *before* it is historical, that there is a *spoken bare life* before someone is made into an exemplar of it. The first Sovereign decision, then, is an act of signification that cuts into undivided life, carving out a space for humans to speak and to understand themselves as temporal beings. When Agamben focuses directly on this structural dimension of Law, acknowledging its fundamental necessity, he appears to arrive at the vanishing point where Foucault's analysis would seem to converge. Only it is not the vantage point at which normative or determinative power seals the deal, as it were, through political techniques and the technology of subjectivization. Sovereign power and subjectivization are part of the process; however, there is an unaccounted-for moment in this process that has nothing (and everything) to do with loosening the normative or totalizing hold of Law on life.

On the contrary, it is here that Agamben preserves and describes, with some inventiveness, the ontological status of, or role for, Law after its tie to normative or determinative Power has been severed. Alleging that there is 'another use of law,' Agamben coins a neologism of sorts (i.e., 'nonrelation') to redeem the politics of this use. Rather than jettisoning Law altogether, Law and life remain joined, but it is a 'nonrelation' that names their connectedness. Law can maintain a 'nonrelation to life' and, in this way, avoid functioning as the Law that acts directly to determine or appropriate the lives, activities, and objects that make up a social world—or the ends to which they are directed and the definite relations that exist between them.[24]

The Law said to enjoy a 'nonrelation to life' is, Agamben contends, a 'pure law'—a law rid of commanding or even referential content and the ends and outcomes that legitimize it. What initiates the political or the human order of politics, for him, is a Law or linguistic entity that refers only to itself, or that is its own activity and nothing else. As Agamben puts it: 'To a word that does not bind, that neither commands nor prohibits anything, but says only itself, would correspond an action as pure means, which shows only itself, without any relation to an end.'[25] This is how a Law becomes pure and an action genuinely political.

The more pure and purified Law becomes, of course, the more difficult it is to map its origins or to see how it might lead to an 'ought' capable of modifying animal or organic existence. Agamben's forbearer here, in an unacknowledged way perhaps, is Kant, who sought out similar reasons to purify Reason; that is, not to restore or revalidate a dogmatism of proper objects, actions, and values, but to turn it, speculatively, back onto itself, to arrive at some conditions for cognition as such. Like Agamben's pure Law, the pure Reason of the first *Critique* 'is in fact occupied only with itself.'[26] What Kant sees as a perversion of Reason is its exercise when determined by an intelligible end, when the chain of causality that determines an action is readily understandable—for example, I do not commit adultery or speak ill of my parents because I have been commanded by God not to do so.

Kant's separation of pure and ordinary Reason, his development of a doctrine and an analytic of 'pure practical reason' seeks precisely to rid human actions and values from their thralldom to the determinative Law of ends. We could say here that politics requires a Law separated from anything straightforwardly or materially relational—in the words of the second *Critique* 'every object of the will (as its determining ground)'[27]—so as to isolate and establish its purity. It is this pure aspect of Law that introduces a break into the ostensibly already-settled questions of why one should act this way and not that, of why these values are legitimate and those not, and so on. The fact that Law is severed from readily understood notions of causality and legitimacy makes it something capable of catalyzing or reminding us of our freedom. As Kant puts it: '[A] will for which the mere lawgiving form of a maxim can alone serve as a law is a free will.'[28] This 'lawgiving' form cannot be 'reasoned out from antecedent data of reason.'[29] Good and evil come only after the Law because, otherwise, it would be the basis for that Law.

Signification as Such

By theorizing Law in this way, Kant and Agamben confront us with (or get us to ask) a very basic question: How can we will something, or make decisions about the lives we life, *un*determined by an intelligible or empirical Law? Who (or what part of the subject) would do this willing? In his famous reading of Freud's 'specimen dream' (i.e., the dream of Irma's injection) in *Seminar II*, Lacan seeks implicitly to address these questions by making more complex the commonplace notion that dreams are 'the disguised fulfillment of repressed wishes'[30]—the staging of illicit desires repressed for immoral or shameful reasons.

In the dream of Irma's injection, Lacan sees something else going on, something much more formal or even philosophical. The key moment of the dream, of course, is the emergence of the formula for trimethylamine—a signifying activity that prevents the subject or agent in the dream (Freud) from merging directly and chaotically with life (down the throat of Irma). Lacan writes: '[J]ust when the world of the dreamer is plunged into the greatest imaginary chaos, discourse [as such] enters into play.'[31] The formula for trimethylamine appears and, at this point, we have, says Lacan, reached the crux of the dream's message, which is nothing less than the very nature of the symbolic order: '[T]here is no other word of the dream than the very nature of the symbolic.'[32] The word passed in the dream is 'a word [that] means nothing except that it is a word'[33]; and this, ultimately, is the formal truth—'the quest for signification as such'[34]—that Lacan discerns beneath Freud's dictum that the scenarios we encounter in our dreams are fulfillments of a wish. That is to say, the deepest wish fulfilled in a dream is the wish to 'pass a certain word.'[35]

This word (and this signifying activity) emerges, quite obviously, from the Unconscious—something logically grasped through its articulations. I am tempted to say here that if there is a political link between Agamben and psychoanalysis on the question of the nonhuman, it rests in the claim that the Unconscious, too, has a 'nonrelation' to life. Which is to say that psychoanalysis, in its insistence on the centrality of the unconscious, cannot but find or delineate a type of nonhuman reality marked by entities that do not simply represent external things but rather what Jean Laplanche calls 'designified-signifiers'.[36] Laplanche's invocation of such signifiers comes in an explicit homage to Lacan, wherein he notes the extent to which passage to the Unconscious is correlative with a loss of referentiality. When a Signifier becomes unconscious, Laplanche suggests, it 'loses its status as presentation (as signifier) in order to become a thing which no longer presents (signifies) anything other than itself.'[37]

What should become clear here is the extent to which, for Lacanian psychoanalysis and for Agamben, the human *does inexorably* maintain a speculative or logically necessary primacy over the nonhuman. Rather than signaling a worrisome recipe for domination, hierarchy, and conflict, the terms and implications of this primacy are the very conditions for politics and a shared world. For both Lacan and Agamben, language is always more than a tool and is used by human beings in ways that are different from other living things. This is because living human beings, in ways they are barely cognizant of, enact the installation of the Signifier in every act of communication—meeting the very material of language *as material* and, in an instant, making it into something meaningful. Before the signifying message of a speech act is the 'quest for signification itself,' and the emergence of a word that wishes only to be a word. As Agamben correctly distinguishes it, this amounts to a dethroning of language:

> It is perhaps time to call into question the prestige that language has enjoyed and continues to enjoy in our culture, as a tool of incomparable potency, efficacy, and beauty. And yet, considered in itself, it is no more beautiful than birdsong, no more efficacious than the signals insects exchange, no more powerful than the roar with which the lion asserts his dominion. The decisive element that confers on human language its peculiar virtue is not the tool itself but the place it leaves to the speaker, in the fact that it prepares within itself a hollowed-out form that the speaker must always assume in order to speak—that is to say, in the ethical relation that is established between the speaker and his language. *The human being is the living being that, in order to speak, must say 'I,' must 'take the word,' assume it and make it his own.*[38]

The place in which the sovereignty of the Signifier leaves the speaker is a gap, a 'hollowed-out' place of fracture and lack.

Avowing the 'peculiar virtue' of human language—a virtue that makes speech acts fundamentally different from the song of birds, the buzzing of insects, the roar of lions—Agamben maintains the Law-executing function of the Signifier in the form of what he calls 'gesture' or an 'event of language.' What gesture communicates is communicability itself; it does not really say something meaningful because a gesture is, for Agamben, 'essentially always a gesture of not being able to figure something out in language.'[39] As an event of language, a gesture performs or repeats what psychoanalysis understands as the installation of the Signifier—something that allows, as Agamben would put it, for the '*factum* of language and the *factum* of community to come to light for an instant.'[40] This is an instant, of course, that forever renders impossible an organic link between the Signifier and a national language or state territory.

Poetry from Guantánamo

To exemplify the basic argument that has been made to this point—that the most authentic and inclusive human community is founded constitutively on the sovereignty of the Signifier—let us now turn to one of the more surprising (and remarkably titled) literary works to be published in the last decade: *Poems from Guantánamo: The Detainees Speak*. There is, of course, much that is disquietingly poignant about the content of the poems that comprise the collection. The poems contain some singular declarations of humiliation and homesickness, despair and sorrow. Many speak directly about having been tortured, about indignities endured during capture and detention (e.g., shackling, not being permitted to void, etc.), and about the absence of loved ones (e.g., parents, spouses, children, etc.). Many of them make desperate appeals to God or to ordinary Americans for freedom and justice.

The very circumstances surrounding the poems' composition, too, are striking. As is well known, detainees were not given the materials necessary for written discourse (e.g., pen, paper, etc.): 'Undeterred, some would draft short poems on Styrofoam cups they had retrieved from their lunch and dinner trays. Lacking writing instruments, they would inscribe their words with pebbles or trace out letters with small dabs of toothpaste, then pass the "cup poems" from cell to cell.'[41] Giving voice to unspeakable suffering and longing, the poems stand alongside the hunger strike as the only forms of rebuke against the Sovereign decree that consigns the prisoner-authors to the state of exception and seeks to reduce their existence to the solitary and animal dimensions of biological life.

What is most salient about these acts of communication, however, is that they take the form of lyric poems, that when 'the detainees speak,' they speak in poetry. This is significant, I think, because lyric poems are unique speech acts that sit astride the threshold that clarifies the human–nonhuman divide. Lyric poems shine a light on this threshold by refusing to conceal entirely the materiality of sound and word that is deployed, manipulated, and aurally or visually arranged. Poems are something quite different from a technical manual, a news report, or most plot-driven narrative prose. These latter forms already assume our status as speaking beings and are thus uninterested in restaging the ontological conditions by which we emerge as creatures of language.

Even as lyric poems foreground their materiality, however, they maintain some tie to meaningful communication, refusing a devolution into babble or nonsense. Versification here has a politics with coordinates in the sovereignty of the Signifier and in the way it enables one to symbolize the material dimension of life—and is itself a material dimension of life—in the very act of negating it. We might say here, in fact, that it is the Sovereign exercise of the Signifier that *creates* the very space for poetry, for a pure *means* of communication that is, momentarily, its own end.

To return to Agamben's terms, poetry shows us the pure Law qua sovereign Signifier. Poetry enacts this law's (or this signifier's) nonrelation to life because what we meet with in poems is the process by which words do not naturally correspond to or determine aspects of life so much as *make possible* a variety of subsequent correspondences or determinations. Against the Law that does seek to determine and secure life, against those sovereignly signifying acts that name and relegate 'enemy combatants' in 'the War on Terror' to the category of the nonhuman, poems remind one of the sovereignty that is *necessarily antecedent to* such an act. This is the sovereignty that is the condition for politics.

It is telling, in this context, that the Pentagon deemed the detainees' poems a security risk, believing them to contain and transmit secret messages. For the Sovereign guardians of security, poems are no different from other instrumental forms of communication; everything about them is tied to their *end*, their hidden or concealed messages. But this is precisely to miss what is so significant about lyric poems, the way their power lies not in (the illusion of) depth or secrecy they contain but rather what happens, in a very elementary way, *on their surface*. We might remember here Martin Heidegger's claim that poems are not like pieces of equipment in which language is used or used up, in which language 'disappears into usefulness.'[42]

The distinction Heidegger introduces between 'projective saying' and 'actual language' is apposite here. Actual language preserves a world of closed (or settled) meanings. For instance, the Arab-Other is the 'enemy combatant' who seeks, by way of terroristic acts of violence, to destroy us and our way of life. The Other is the barbaric animal who must either become a friend or be destroyed altogether. Projective saying, however, is what 'prepar[es] the sayable'; it 'simultaneously brings the unsayable as such into a world.'[43]

Consider the enjambment that distinguishes the second and sixth stanzas of Abdullah Thani Faris Al Anazi's poem, 'To My Father.' In the first stanza, the poem's speaker names the anguished homesickness he experiences, having been incarcerated at Guantánamo for two years. The poem conveys just what the speaker is separated from—from the traditional application of kohl to the eyes, from fields of 'lavender cotton,' and from the togetherness of time spent in the homes of family members. Al Anazi's poem contains a directive, and he imagines it reaching its intended audience and producing a gesture by proxy, as it were. That gesture is a kiss of the speaker's father's forehead: 'Kiss him on the forehead, for he is my father/Fate has divided us, like the parting of a parent from a/newborn.'

In the sixth stanza, the speaker's address is directly to a God 'who governs creation with providence' and who is deservedly worshipped. To this God, Al Anazi addresses a kind of prayerful appeal: 'Grant serenity to a heart that beats with oppression./And release this prisoner from the tight bonds of/confinement.' Both stanzas end with single words—'newborn' and 'confinement'—that have been separated from the poetic declarations to which they belong. In meeting these single words on separate lines, we meet with the capacity of poems to signify the *very act of signifying*.

The single word reminds us, for an instant, that words are things before we are made to see, too, that words are always more than mere things. In this case, their arrangement on the page—or their separation by an extra breath from the words that precede them—enables one to reenact a movement from organic or animal life to the properly human world of language. The pure discernment of the word gives way, in an instant, to 'figuring out' what the speech act seeks to convey—the pain of separation from loved ones and the barbarism of Guantánamo's prison conditions.

The lesson of the poem—and perhaps of lyric poetry itself—is that the only way to oppose the outrage of a historically Sovereign power and its relegation of human beings to the category of the nonhuman is with sovereign Power itself or as such. From the historically created state of exception, the detainees speak. And they, like the rest of us, speak poems.

Notes

1. Giorgio Agamben, *Homo Sacer: Sovereign Power and Bare Life*, trans. Daniel Heller-Roazen (Stanford: Stanford University Press, 1998), p. 5.
2. Foucault rejects the view that sees the Individual as the victim of Power, or its possible adversary. Power is not 'applied to' individuals, who either accept or oppose it. Rather, power has already, in a sense, 'passed through' individuals, who are its 'relays.' As Foucault puts it, it is 'a mistake to think of the individual as a sort of elementary nucleus, a primitive atom or some multiple, inert matter to which power is applied, or which is struck by a power that subordinates or destroys individuals. In actual fact, one of the first effects of power is that it allows bodies, gestures, discourses, and desires to be identified and constituted as something individual. The individual is not, in other words, power's opposite number; the individual is one of power's first effects' (Michel Foucault, 'Society Must Be Defended.' In*: Lectures at the Collège de France, 1975–1976*, trans. David Macey (New York: Picador, 2003), 29–30).
3. Agamben (1998), p. 6.
4. Ibid.
5. Ibid., p. 8.
6. Ibid.
7. For the penultimate American instance of this, recall Frederick Douglass' poignant account of an overseer's killing of a slave named Demby and the conclusion Douglass draws from it: 'I speak advisedly when I say this—that killing a slave, or any colored person, in Talbot country, Maryland, is not treated as a crime, either by the courts or by the community' (Frederick Douglass, *Narrative of the Life of Frederick Douglass* [New York: Oxford, 2009], p. 32).
8. See here Foucault's contention that the very emergence of Biology as a scientific discipline is synchronous with the invention of life. Prior to the middle of the eighteenth century, he writes, 'biology was unknown' for the 'very simple reason…that life itself did not exist' (Michel Foucault, *The Order of Things*, trans. Alan Sheridan [New York: Random House, 1994)] pp. 127–128).
9. Michel Foucault, *The History of Sexuality: An Introduction, Vol. I*, trans. Robert Hurley (New York: Random House, 1990), p. 142.
10. Foucault (2003), p. 25.
11. Agamben (1998), p. 11.

12. Ibid., p. 26.
13. Jacques Lacan, *The Seminar of Jacques Lacan, Book XX: Encore, 1972–1973,* trans. Bruce Fink (New York: Norton, 1998), p. 3.
14. Richard L. Rubenstein, *The Cunning of History: The Holocaust and the American Future* (New York: Harper and Row, 1987), p. 87.
15. Agamben (1998), p. 59.
16. The esteem in which Agamben holds the Franciscans has its coordinates here, since the Franciscans 'actualize' a 'neutralization of law with respect to life' (Giorgio Agamben, *The Highest Poverty: Monastic Rules and Form-of-Life*, trans. Adam Kotsko (Stanford: Stanford University Press, 2013), p. 111. The Franciscans enact a radical reclamation of life, 'subtract[ing] life from the sphere of law.' From this standpoint, a kind of radical freedom is said to reside in the dissolution of the very distinction between human and nonhuman, between political and biological/animal life. There is no shortage of contemporary examples of the ostensible pleasures to be had when we have freed ourselves from Law and the values and hierarchies and pathologies it erects. See, for example, the phenomenon of Zoosexuality, which revalues sex with—or a sexual orientation toward—nonhuman animals as part of 'a loving inter-species relationship' (Samantha Hurn, *Humans and Other Animals: Cross-cultural Perspectives on Human-Animal Interactions* [London: Pluto Press, 2012], p. 193).
17. Gerald Bruns, *On Ceasing to Be Human* (Stanford: Stanford University Press, 2011). Bruns finds in Foucault a version or incarnation of sovereignty that escapes symbolization entirely—someone 'perhaps no longer human, neither human nor nonhuman but a figure of alterity without reference to the same' (pp. 28–29). For Bruns, Foucault radically rejects all normative constrictions. He writes that Foucault is 'someone who thinks that we are capable of "practicing" freedom as an essentially anarchic form of life. An anarchic form of life enjoys a shortfall of criteria; it is one in which nothing is settled in advance, and the idea is to keep things (and oneself) in motion' (p. 50).
18. Agamben (1998), p. 21.
19. G.W.F. Hegel, *Phenomenology of Spirit*, trans. A. V. Miller (New York: Oxford University Press, 1977), p. 66.
20. G.W.F. Hegel, *Science of Logic*, trans. A. V. Miller (Atlantic Highlands, NJ: Humanities Press International, 1989), p. 45.

21. G.W.F. Hegel, *The Encyclopaedia Logic: Part I of the Encyclopaedia of the Philosophical Sciences*, trans. T. F. Garaets, W. A. Suchting, and H. S. Harris (Indianapolis: Hackett, 1991), p. 152.
22. Ibid., p. 762.
23. Catherine Malabou, *The Future of Hegel: Plasticity, Temporality and Dialectic*, trans. Lisabeth During (New York Routledge, 2005), p. 68.
24. As Marx well knew, Law inaugurates a relationship between an object and the whole: 'A cotton-spinning jenny is a machine for spinning cotton. Only in certain circumstances does it become capital. Torn from those circumstances it is no more capital than gold is money or sugar the price of sugar.' (Karl Marx, *Wage-Labor, and Capital*, trans. Harriet E. Lothrop [New York: New York Labor News Company, 1902], 35). See also, in this regard, Lukács' contention that 'the intelligibility of objects develops in proportion as we grasp their function in the totality to which they belong' (Georg Lukács, *History and Class Consciousness*, trans, Rodney Livingstone [Cambridge, Mass.: MIT Press, 1971], 13).
25. Giorgio Agamben, *State of Exception*, trans. Kevin Attell (Chicago: University of Chicago Press, 2005), p. 88.
26. Immanuel Kant, *Critique of Pure Reason*, trans. Werner S. Pluhar (Indianapolis: Hackett Publishing Company, 1996), p. 645.
27. Immanuel Kant, *Critique of Practical Reason*, trans. Lewis White Beck, 3rd edition (Upper Saddle River, NJ: Prentice Hall, 1993), p. 160.
28. Ibid., p. 162.
29. Ibid., p. 164.
30. Sigmund Freud, *Five Lectures on Psycho-Analysis*, trans. James Strachey (New York: W.W. Norton, 1977), p. 36.
31. Jacques Lacan, *The Seminar of Jacques Lacan, Book II: The Ego in Freud's Theory and in the Technique of Psychoanalysis, 1954–1955*, trans. Sylvana Tomaselli (New York: W. W. Norton, 1991), p. 170.
32. Ibid., p. 160.
33. Ibid., p. 170.
34. Ibid., p. 160.
35. Ibid., p. 126.
36. Jean Laplanche, 'A Short Treatise on the Unconscious,' *Essays on Otherness* (New York: Routledge, 2003), 92.
37. Ibid., p. 90.
38. Giorgio Agamben, *The Sacrament of Language: An Archeology of the Oath*, trans. Adam Kotsko (Stanford: Stanford University Press, 2011), p. 71.

39. Giorgio Agamben, *Means Without End: Notes on Politics*, trans. Vincenzo Binetti and Cesare Casarino (Minneapolis: University of Minnesota Press, 2004), p. 59.
40. Ibid., p. 70.
41. Marc Falkoff, 'Notes on Guantánamo.' In *Poems from Guantánamo: The Detainees Speak* (Iowa City: Iowa University Press, 2007), p. 3.
42. Martin Heidegger, 'The Origin of the Work of Art.' In *Poetry, Language, Thought*, trans, Albert Hofstadter (New York: Harper and Row, 1971), p. 46.
43. Ibid., p. 74.

Bibliography

Agamben, Giorgio. 1998. *Homo Sacer: Sovereign Power and Bare Life*. Trans. Daniel Heller-Roazen. Stanford: Stanford University Press.

———. 2004. *Means Without End: Notes on Politics*. Trans. Vincenzo Binetti and Cesare Casarino. Minneapolis: University of Minnesota Press.

———. 2005. *State of Exception*. Trans. Kevin Attell. Chicago: University of Chicago Press.

———. 2011. *The Sacrament of Language: An Archeology of the Oath*. Trans. Adam Kotsko. Stanford: Stanford University Press.

———. 2013. *The Highest Poverty: Monastic Rules and Form-of-Life*. Trans. Adam Kotsko. Stanford: Stanford University Press.

Bruns, Gerald. 2011. *On Ceasing to Be Human*. Stanford: Stanford University Press.

Douglass, Frederick. 2009. *Narrative of the Life of Frederick Douglass*. New York: Oxford.

Falkoff, Marc. 2007. Notes on Guantánamo. In *Poems from Guantánamo: The Detainees Speak*. Iowa City: Iowa University Press.

Foucault, Michel. 1990. *The History of Sexuality: An Introduction, Vol. I*. Trans. Robert Hurley. New York: Random House.

———. 1994. *The Order of Things*. Trans. Alan Sheridan. New York: Random House.

———. 2003. Society Must Be Defended. *Lectures at the Collège de France, 1975–1976*. Trans. David Macey. New York: Picador.

Freud, Sigmund. 1977. *Five Lectures on Psycho-Analysis*. Trans. James Strachey. New York: W. W. Norton.

Hegel, G.W.F. 1977. *Phenomenology of Spirit*. Trans. A. V. Miller. New York: Oxford University Press.

———. 1989. *Science of Logic*. Trans. A. V. Miller. Atlantic Highlands: Humanities Press International.

———. 1991. *The Encyclopaedia Logic: Part I of the Encyclopaedia of the Philosophical Sciences*. Trans. T. F. Garaets, W. A. Suchting, and H. S. Harris. Indianapolis: Hackett.

Heidegger, Martin. 1971. The Origin of the Work of Art. In *Poetry, Language, Thought*. Trans. Albert Hofstadter. New York: Harper and Row.

Hurn, Samantha. 2012. *Humans and Other Animals: Cross-Cultural Perspectives on Human-Animal Interactions*. London: Pluto Press.

Kant, Immanuel. 1993. *Critique of Practical Reason*. Trans. Lewis White Beck, 3rd ed. Upper Saddle River: Prentice Hall.

———. 1996. *Critique of Pure Reason*. Trans. Werner S. Pluhar. Indianapolis: Hackett.

Lacan, Jacques. 1991. *The Seminar of Jacques Lacan, Book II: The Ego in Freud's Theory and in the Technique of Psychoanalysis, 1954–1955*. Trans. Sylvana Tomaselli. New York: Norton.

———. 1998. *The Seminar of Jacques Lacan, Book XX: Encore, 1972–1973*. Trans. Bruce Fink. New York: Norton.

Laplanche, Jean. 2003. A Short Treatise on the Unconscious. In *Essays on Otherness*, ed. John Fletcher. New York: Routledge.

Lukàcs, Georg. 1971. *History and Class Consciousness: Studies in Marxist Dialectics*. Trans. Rodney Livingstone. Cambridge: MIT Press.

Rubenstein, Richard L. 1987. *The Cunning of History: The Holocaust and the American Future*. New York: Harper and Row.

Part II

Applications

Triplicity in Spencer-Brown, Lacan, and Poe

Don Kunze

When speculative realists argue that objects—and objectivity itself—should be considered apart from subjects and subjectivities, they recommend a mathematical approach, but what kind of mathematics? Levi Bryant's *The Democracy of Objects* provides a specific and representative answer when he takes his project of 'onticology' to George Spencer-Brown's Boolean calculus in *Laws of Form*. This non-numerical notation uses a single symbol, ˥, an angle—alternatively called a 'cross' or 'call'—that divides space into an unmarked region surrounded by a marked space outside.[1]

At the same time the mark divides space, it indicates what it contains within its concave mark. Bryant makes an important distinction at this point. He claims that because indications interact with, represent, or point at something 'in the world,' a function of indication follows the more primary function of distinction. Bryant argues that this is the natural order of things, evident from the fact that the indication that the sun

D. Kunze (✉)
Pennsylvania State University, State College, PA, USA

G. Basu Thakur, J.M. Dickstein (eds.), *Lacan and the Nonhuman*,
The Palgrave Lacan Series, DOI 10.1007/978-3-319-63817-1_8

is shining requires an *implicit binary distinction* between light and darkness. Binary first; then indication, pointing at something 'in the world,' comes second.

Bryant represents this as Spencer-Brown's position on the matter.[2] But, this does not tally with what Spencer-Brown himself wrote in his *Laws of Form*: 'We take as given the idea of a distinction and the idea of an indication, and that it is not possible to make an indication without drawing a distinction.'[3] Possibly, one could read this as meaning 'without *first* drawing a distinction.' Nonetheless, Louis Kauffman, Spencer-Brown's leading advocate in the United States, has on many occasions emphasized that indication and distinction are simultaneous: '[T]here can be no mark without a distinction and there can be no distinction without indication…*the act of distinction is necessarily circular.* …The act of drawing a distinction involves a circulation as in drawing a circle, or moving back and forth between two states.'

What does this mean, and why is it important? My intention is to show how Kaufmann's point is revealingly Lacanian. At the same time, I hope to convince object-oriented ontologists (OOO) what they might learn from a deeper consideration of Freudian–Lacanian psychoanalysis. This aim goes beyond critiquing Bryant's use of Spencer-Brown's calculus. It requires a thematic reorganization of thinking around the concept of 'thirdness' or 'triplicity,' the movement from binaries to self-referencing and self-generating capabilities within the Symbolic—*automata* that can be found in the merger of Form and Content implicit in *Laws of Form*.

The Kauffman–Spencer-Brown slogan, 'self-reference and reference are intimately intertwined,' echoes Lacan's argument about *triplicity* in relation to metalanguage.[4] Spencer-Brown recognizes Form as a 'self-awareness' that goes past the (Boolean) binary of appearances versus realities. Lacan's version of this addresses the problem of having to talk about language (the Symbolic) with language (language theory). Pierre Skriabine summarizes Lacan's position: 'There is no metalanguage… because the Other of the Other does not exist; there is only a barred Other [represented by the *matheme* Ⱥ, for ~~*Autre*~~, '~~Other~~'], marked by inconsistency or incompleteness.'[5]

To solve this duplicity problem, Lacan creates a triplicity through the addition of the idea of 'ex-sistence,' the status of the category of the Real, which supplements the 'appearances' of the Imaginary and the 'realities' of the Symbolic through conditions of absence, negation, and lack.[6] Lacan's *matheme* for the Signifier of the lack in the Other, S(Ⱥ), is the defect *within* the Symbolic's signifying chains that 'extimates' an Otherness that 'ex-sists' rather than 'exists.' Spencer-Brown echoes this in his insistence that Form is 'self-aware' because it includes the *means* of representing within the grammar of representing.

In providing an appearance–reality counterpart to Lacan's extimation of an ex-sisting Otherness, Spencer-Brown, I would claim, outspeculates speculative realists and nearly out-Lacans Lacan when he says that 'there can be no appearance that is not an awareness of appearance and, of course, no awareness that is not an appearance of awareness.'[7] This is a deep-space version of the axiomatic *coincidence of distinction* (appearance of awareness) and *indication* (awareness of distinction)—that is, CDI. Spencer-Brown replaces the duplicity of scientific doctrine based on the binary of appearance–reality with a triplicity that reveals, beneath his Boolean calculus, a pre- or non-Boolean basis. That Lacan's resistance to the idea of a metalanguage involves pre- or non-Boolean stratagems nearly identical, or at least sympathetic to Spencer-Brown's, is both striking and indicative.[8]

'Triplicity' refers to the necessity that the Symbolic create and then rely on a zone *outside* of itself, correlated to an *internal* defect, gap, or lack. This 'action at a distance,' this *entanglement*, associated with metonymy rather than metaphor, constitutes a form of 'vertical meaning' in relation to the 'horizontal' signifying chains of the Symbolic (Fig. 1). Its indica-

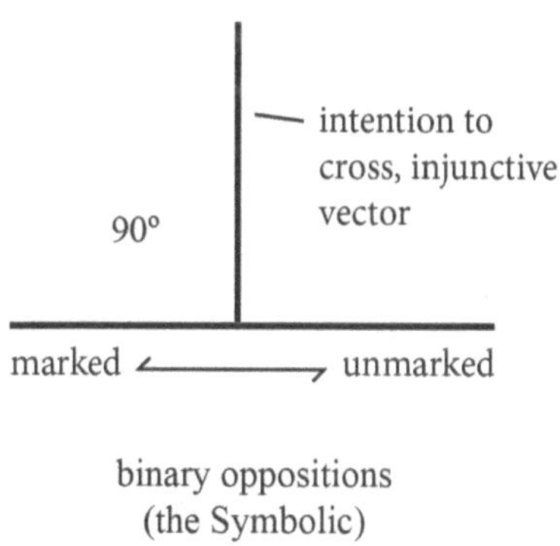

Fig. 1 The 'horizontal' signifying chains of the Symbolic intersect orthogonally at the point of a gap with a 'vertical' injunctive that constitutes a vector by which the Form may reenter itself

tion function is embodied as an *injunction to cross* a boundary distinguishing two spaces, where one space contains representations concluding with an 'unmarked empty space' and the other contains 'containing.'

What is this metonymic zone outside of itself correlative to the defect within the Symbolic? Louis Armand suggests that it is none other than the world without the subject, not only 'post-humanist' but the *posthuman* world, 'from which man has disappeared.' Citing Lacan's 1954 seminar on the technics of the mirror dialectic, Armand calls attention to Lacan's strange invention of a 'Cartesian cybernetics, an ego *ex machina*,' in contrast to Walter Benjamin's famous 1937 essay, 'The Work of Art in the Age of Mechanical Reproduction.' '[I]t is precisely the camera, as a mechanism of the gaze, by means of which Lacan envisages a certain "aura" *as affecting itself*, as we shall see' [emphasis mine]:

> ...[T]here remains only this mechanical form of reflexivity: a camera alone in nature. The 'presence' of this camera is made to 'mirror,' in a sense, the non-presence of man. At the same time, an actual mirror, although we are not told this (we expect it), is itself 'in' the camera, while the camera itself is trained on the surface of a lake, in which there appears an inverted image of a mountain. And despite, as Lacan says, 'all living beings having disappeared, the camera can nonetheless record the image of the mountain in the lake,' which is thus also (paradoxically) a record of its non-presence there.[9]

In the triplicity that is not just 'post-binary' but 'post-human' as well, Boolean logic breaks down to reveal its self-automating, self-referential, 'self-extimating' machine structure 'detached from the activity of the subject,' which Lacan identifies as the Symbolic. 'Post-human' automation had already been evident in Joyce's *Finnegans Wake*, in what Armand calls 'a like process of autoproduction and topical recursion (symptomatisation), in which the plagiarist-author figure of Shem-the-Penman is depicted as writing his name in "shit encaustic"' across the entire surface of his body. Mixing *topos* with *tropos* and *copros*, Shem writes his own name 'in a single act of "reflexivity" or autopoiesis (the retroverted *nom-du-Père* whose metonym—*nom-du-fils*—is a "coprophagic" counterpart, *à la Artaud*.'[10] Triplicity is an autonomous, self-referential writing machine.[11]

For Spencer-Brown, triplicity is the necessity of including the observer in the observed, radically, at the level of the calculus: 'An observer, since he distinguishes the space he occupies, is also a mark. …We see how that the first distinction, the mark, and the observer are not only interchangeable, but [also], in the form, identical.'[12] Then, because the mathematician–observer is not describing a sunset or anything else in the spatiotemporal landscape but rather is specifying an *injunction*, an action, the indication that *necessarily* accompanies distinction indicates action, not the kind of 'pictorial' condition based on a binary distinction that Bryant appears to suggest.

If we compare Lacan's 'thirdness of the Real' to Spencer-Brown's 'thirdness of injunction,' we can see the logic behind CDI—the coincidence of distinction (appearance of awareness) and indication (awareness of appearance). The Real amounts to an act that follows a binary impasse and is in some ways the password that is enacted in a register outside of language's normal semantic functions. Thirdness as action recalls Lacan's treatment of the dilemma of the Three Prisoners, who must decide whether the dot pinned on their backs is one of two black dots or three white dots in the warden's collection.

Robert Samuels summarized the prisoners' response in terms of a tripartite temporality.[13] Because all three prisoners have white dots, the first temporality is the *moment* each prisoner, without knowing what his two fellow inmates see, perceives two white dots. The second temporality is a 'time of understanding,' structured by the binary of having *either* a black *or* a white dot. The third is the moment of concluding. All three prisoners realize that their colleagues would have moved immediately if they had seen a black dot but *instead have hesitated.* Once this hesitation registers *simultaneously*, all three prisoners rush for the door.

The time of understanding is closest to what we might call 'normal time,' dominated by the binary of knowing–not-knowing, visibility–invisibility. This is the time of the ticking clock, of anxiety aimed forward and memory backward. The key point is that this binary time is sandwiched between two 'non-time times,' the moment of seeing only white dots (but not knowing that all see them) and the instantaneous rush to the door propelled by the retroactive realization of the meaning of hesitation.

This time triplet seems to invite consideration of C. S. Peirce's thirdness—a 'product of an interpretive *pro*-ject.' This product is an *act*. So, when Spencer-Brown calls 'indication' an *injunction*, we think of the Real of Lacan. This is the Real of absence, the lack, that enjoins a temporality that, in Spencer-Brown fashion, *moves past* any 'picture of the situation,' any 'contextualizing' of place or time, to an identification connecting the mark and the maker of the mark, the subject and the Signifier of its deficient construction, the Other, S(Ⱥ).

There are two spooky coincidences that connect Lacan and Spencer-Brown. First is the coincidence of Spencer-Brown's and Lacan's determination to critique scientific 'duplicity' and, further, to specify a thirdness around the idea of construction and retroactive temporality. Second, both Spencer-Brown and Lacan connect their thirdnesses to a knowledge that lies outside of the 'flat' or 'horizontal' Symbolic but within the 'project' of theory in the form of *automaton*. For Lacan, this is the unconscious's perfect memory: How, according to Bruce Fink, the unconscious 'topologically' maintains both (1) grammatical rules excluding incorrect combinations and (2) an internal totalizing-accumulative 'trash pile' that has *no need of any subject whatsoever*—an *automaton*.[14]

Thirdness for Spencer-Brown critically depends on the simultaneity and circularity of distinction and indication, CDI, where *automaton* is found in the re-entry of the Form into itself.[15] Lacan's exteriorized thirdness, the category of the Real that indicates the discovery of a password written in a 'parallel register' to escape the Symbolic, identifies (= discovers the escape route connecting) the 'interior' of the prison with the 'outside' of the construction of the puzzle. The bounded space thus is escaped in an act that, in Spencer-Brown fashion, identifies the maker with the mark, J = ~J.

In opposition to Bryant's delay of indication as 'interpretation afforded by binary distinction,' Spencer-Brown and Lacan both appear to agree that distinction's coincidence with indication is not simply labeling spaces that have been divided, but an unconscious *self-awareness* that works in the absence of the subject; and that the *automatism* is required to move from the 'flat space' of demonstration to topological spaces, where self-reference can be understood through recursive structures (e.g., the Möbius band, cross-cap, and Klein bottle).

Spencer-Brown asserts that, to maintain consistency of his axiomatic interactions of marked and unmarked spaces, one must presume that the surface of demonstration is flat; however, then he opens the way to a 'corrected' phenomenology of contradiction once the outside marked space is allowed to be curved, and the form is able to 're-enter' itself.[16] For Lacan, curvature gets past the dialectic opposition of elements that are contradictory on the surface of the 'something,' which will be relatable in a space (and time) of nothing.[17]

Bryant would center Spencer-Brown's calculus on its purely Boolean ability to distinguish and thus overemphasize the binary contradictions and the flatness of their surface of demonstration. But if, in the spirit of Kauffman, CDI extends the calculus toward questions of self-reference, recursion, and trans- or pre-Boolean functions, the calculus shows how the idea of triplicity is the necessary critical-theory complement to binary distinctions and phenomenological–positivistic duplicity of appearance–reality. Indication, in its thirdness, is this supplement. Lacan writes indication in terms of the unconscious, and Spencer-Brown prefers the minor key of identity of opposites, J = ~J. Both expose a stranger truth about thirdness: *automaton*.

The Lipogram and the Perpendicular Player

In Georges Perec's famous lipogram novel, *A Void*, the text tells stories in a seemingly normal way, but entirely without words containing the letter 'e.' The reader begins to notice strange diversions and eddy currents ('clinamen') in the narrative flow, and where convention should dominate, Perec's circumlocutions to construct 'non-e' ways of writing finally give away the secret.[18] The reader himself or herself has unconsciously created metaleptic meaning effects based on the absence—'something has come of nothing,' to quote Spencer-Brown's *Laws of Form*—and it is imperative to ask whether the emergence of this something owes to the thirdness of distinction and indication coincidence, where indication takes on the role of the external–internal 'vertical' vector shown earlier in Fig. 1.

Such presence of absence is the focus of Lacan's analysis of another text dealing with the absence of a letter, this time the kind of 'letter' that has a destination in Lacanian terms, the basis of Edgar Allen Poe's short story, 'The Purloined Letter.' As most readers will know, an unnamed Minister D--, to gain control over the Queen of France, steals a letter that would create a scandal if made known to the King. The minister hides it in his apartment with the simple ruse of leaving it out in the open, where the police, acting for the Queen, will least expect to find it.

Lacan notes: 'For [the police's] imbecility is…the imbecility of the realist who does not pause to observe that nothing, however deep into the bowels of the world a hand may shove it, will ever be hidden there, since *another hand* can retrieve it' [emphasis mine].[19] The imbecility of the realist is represented by its *interior* journey inside the original mark; while the genius of Dupin, Poe explains, is that he engages the role played by the point of view (POV) by retroactively realizing the *exterior* of the mark—where the mark *coincides precisely* with the indication of *its own* space of demonstration/representation and realizes a thirdness of identity past the hide-and-seek binary.

Poe himself notes this identity function: 'The boy [who] won all the marbles of the school…had some principle of guessing; and this lay in mere observation and admeasurement of the astuteness of his opponents.'[20] This reference to Morra, the game of odds and evens, points to the issue of how binaries operate not just in the plane of representation but between the frame and its implied POV. Although binaries of the either/or variety lie flat in the plane of representation, as so many 'lefts and rights' of a given condition, Poe's 'admeasurement of the astuteness of [one's] opponents' is logically independent from, and graphically orthogonal to, this binary of hide-and-seek.

Admeasurement of one's opponent erects a graphic standpoint above the entire plane of representation, a POV line metaphorically placing the player perpendicular to the played (again, see Fig. 1). This is 'indication'—awareness of appearance—in its purest and most radical form. Its super-dimensional status is transferred to the concavity of the mark on the page. Poe signals this inside of the story by referring to 'odd' and 'even' in other senses, as 'unusual,' 'equal,' or even 'evening.' The story takes place, after all, on an 'odd evening.'

The addition of the dimension of the POV of the 'perpendicular player' is the topological equivalent of self-reference (Fig. 2), where indication

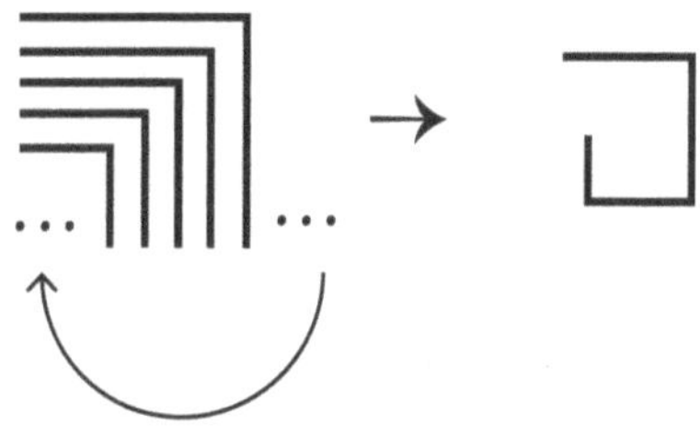

Fig. 2 Concentric marks ('consecution') lead to an interior concavity of marks within marks, where, as Dupin comments, the 'hand that conceals' is forever foiled by the 'hand that finds.' When concentricity moves outward, however, the space of the POV is engaged, and with it the topological/recursive position, which, when accessed, engages the dimension of time

and distinction are coincident once the innermost space of interiorizing concentricity is 'found' by the new $n + 1$—the outermost point, the view of which has trumped that of its 'opponent.' Its astuteness gains it access to the innermost frame. The theme of the palindrome, reverse reading, reinforces the theme of the lipogram.

Dupin knows the hiding place because he 'knows' the Minister to be his palindromic twin, and even the hiding place is a phonetic palindrome ('card-rack' = 'kcar-drak'). The palindrome converts dimensions to vectors in order to open up a *double channel* linking left with right and, thus, disguises/occults the negation. Lacan says: 'To purloin is thus *mettre de côté* (to set aside) or … *mettre à gauche* (to put to the left side…and to tuck away).'[21] Adjusting to Spencer-Brown's way of writing marks with the unmarked innermost space to the left, we say in following this convention, 'to put to the *right* side,' with the benefit that this switch emphasizes how the Minister's point of view is 'a-*droit*-ly' folded into the plane of representation to create a double channel, occulting invisibility within visibility (Fig. 3).[22]

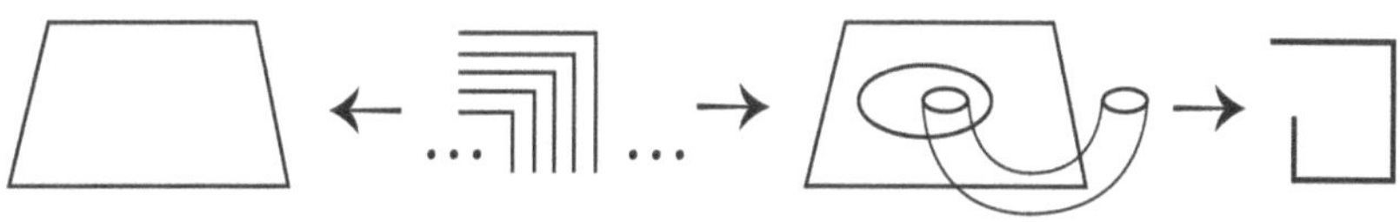

Fig. 3 While the police go *left*, Dupin goes *right*. Dupin's method (like Poe's) is a version of the game of Morra

Lacan begins his essay on 'The Purloined Letter' with a reference to repetition compulsion. How would this play out in the onto-topology of the calculus? Concavity of the mark makes the interior of demonstration into a *mise-en-abîme*, the bad infinities of which convert into an onto-topology that corrects this infinite regress by enclosing the whole expression with an external frame. The result is, in Spencer-Brown's terms, 're-entry into the form'; in Lacan's terms, this is extimity (i.e., *extimité*). Considered as a circuit, linearity versus nonlinearity can be compared to paired inverter gates that regulate a perfect division between positive and negative states (Fig. 4, *left*). A single inverter gate, however, causes a passing signal to oscillate, 1→0→1→0→1→0… (Fig. 4, *right*).

Oscillation of the circuit functionally returns energy to the gate, which, as a 'pure binary,' *cannot* distinguish between inside/outside, subject/object, left/right. Identity, Kauffman explains, is the same as confusing one thing with another. The '=' means 'is indistinguishable from.'[23] Dupin 'equates' the concealed space of the letter with the open display position of the card-rack. The circuit of the story returns the 'left' of concealment to the 'right' of discovery.

Lacan's example of the 'technique of the ostrich' inspires one to characterize the death drive circuit in optical terms: 'the way in which subjects, owing to their displacement, relay each other in the course of the intersubjective repetition…[thanks to] the place that a pure signifier—the purloined letter—comes to occupy' in a trio (for Lacan: the Queen, the Minister, and Dupin).[24] In my version I would substitute, for the Queen, the *invisibility* of her letter, which, as purloined (i.e.,

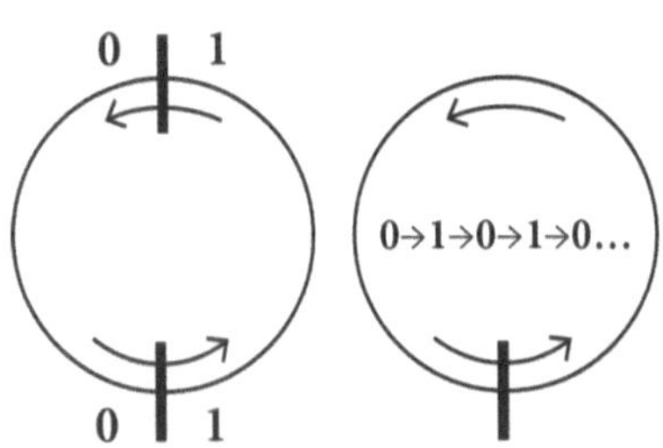

Fig. 4 Paired inverter gates (*left*) ensure permanent distribution of values in the circuit, while a single inverter gate (*right*) causes a passing signal to oscillate

set-aside), Lacan aptly identifies as a 'pure signifier.' Second would be the term *blindness*, which the Minister creates by leaving the letter out in the open. My third term would be the operation of *theft*, more specifically, theft-by-stealth—the 'Dupin function.'

The justification for these substitutions, I propose, is the way 'blindness' and 'invisibility' must form a dyad to allow for the pickpocket's art of 'body loading'—creation of numbness around the victim's body to facilitate the entry of the hand and the exit of goods.[25] Because invisibility is on the side of the object and blindness is on the side of the subject, the dyad's symmetry 'works the perpendicular' to accomplish re-entry into the form, the primitive cultural counterpart of which is theft by stealth.

The 3-Monster: The trinity is the composite subject, which can be viewed as a divinatory sign, a *monstrum*, in the same way that the 'chimera,' with the lion's head, the goat's body, and the serpent's tale, was really a fable about the mysterious *temporal* conjunction of seasons in the annual cycle. 'Optical monstrosity' here means the blindness of the one, the (illusion of) invisibility of the second, and the theft-by-stealth of the third. The inverter gate, the 'Dupin function,' converts/inverts blindness and invisibility, allowing the circuit to *steal* from the one to *return* to the other.

Because Spencer-Brown's mark is concave, the *mise-en-abîme* of the 'invisible' letter becomes susceptible to the theft-by-stealth of the detective who stands 'at one remove from a fool'—the Minister—while the Minister is made to *look away* at the moment of theft.[26] Dupin enacts the coincidence of distinction and indication when he 'crosses the line' between invisibility and blindness to fool the poet-mathematician Minister. His '=' ('failure to observe a distinction' in the sense of failing to notice a 'no trespassing' sign) is the point of Lacanian *extimité*, which we can locate at the inverter gate of the 101, 010… cycle shown earlier in Fig. 4. Whether the lipogram is a missing 'e' or a letter that will eventually reach the Queen, we recognize that the 'something that comes of nothing' does not simply come; it must be stolen—stolen by stealth (i.e., by art)—and that this kind of theft-by-stealth requires a particular kind of thief, a Hermes able to confer the power of the secret on what is stolen.[27]

The Optical Monstrosity of Sorites

An astute Poe scholar, Richard Kopley, demonstrated how 'The Purloined Letter' benefits from a chiastic lambda (Λ) structure, where eight paired statements frame the center of the story.[28] In some cases, the pairs are perfect mirror images, as in the chiastic inversion, 'all fools are poets' and 'all poets are fools.' The pairings pile up the story toward the apex of the Λ, where Dupin produces the previously invisible letter in exchange for the reward money—itself a chiastic trade. Between the separated pairs, the story itself constructs a 'reader's lipogram' in that the linear reader, like the police in the story, cannot see the purloined space framed by symmetrical elements, even though these echoes are set out in plain view.

'The Purloined Letter' pairs statements to create a flip point, a chiastic mirror. The echo chamber created by the delays separating the pairs frames this optical function with precision. The invisible letter is made visible in the *moment* Dupin produces it out of an invisible nowhere, a moment that is expanded as the basis of the story of how that same invisibility is engineered within the logic of the left–right game of Morra.[29]

Lacan does not mention this lipogram ploy, but it would seem to fit in nicely with (1) his own 'thirdness' (the addition of a demonstration of numerical sequences, attached to the main Poe critique); (2) the idea of a Real that constitutes an externality for the appearance–reality binary of the Imaginary and Symbolic; and (3) the here-but-not-here status of Poe's own supplement of the mystery story's narrative (i.e., an elaboration about the chirality of the game of Morra)—Poe's triplicity added to the duplicity of the appearance versus the reality hide-and-seek game. When Spencer-Brown makes it clear that his thirdness holds the key to the 'Eigenform,' a pre-Boolean way of getting past appearance–reality duplicity, we are invited to compare the Lacanian Real to a combined solution that is subject-free in both mathematical and psychoanalytic terms. Is not this what speculative realists are looking for?

Near the end of the book, *Laws of Form*, Spencer-Brown shows off a bit by using calculus notation to solve—with astonishing speed—one of Lewis Carroll's sorites puzzles.[30] To give away the secret of how Carroll constructed these, it is first necessary to pay respect to the idea of sorites. It is the process of gradual accumulation or attrition: How grains of sand fall one by one, to the point that they become a pile; or how the hairs of a balding man disappear one by one, until his head becomes bald. The processes are gradual; however, the *moment* the idea of a sand pile or bald head comes into focus is accompanied by a *retroactive realization* that the 'pile' or the 'bald head' had already been in place before that moment of recognition, not just as a predecessor but also as an efficient cause. This is analogous to the prisoners' rush to the door after realizing the meaning of their mutual *delay*—which we as readers of Poe's story do when we realize the delay of the Λ chiasmus. Without revealing the formal name for this 'one grain more' logic, Žižek has ascribed it as nothing less than the logic of (Hegelian) emergence: How necessity arises out of pure contingency.[31]

Carroll's puzzles are made up of an even number of statements paired in mirrored versions (Fig. 5) so that an odd couple will remain as the 'answer,' even though the 'answer' concept is not known as such until retroactive realization occurs; it is the remainder. Each orphan appears as predicat*ed* and predicat*ing*. One term of each pair is inside the concave distinguishing mark, ⏋; the other is outside. When all the paired mirror-terms are 'canceled out,' only two orphans will be left; each orphan appears only once, one as predicat*ing*, the other as predicat*ed*. Combined, they constitute the answer to the puzzle.

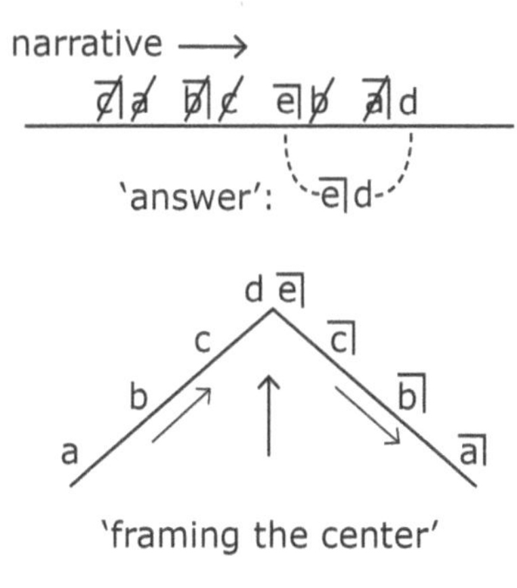

Fig. 5 In the sorites of Lewis Carroll's puzzles, all elements but two appear twice, in mirroring forms. The terms and their 'echoes' frame the middle of the story, the exchange of 'the purloined letter' for the reward check

It is easy to see that the 'pivot' of Lewis Carroll's sorites works as the 'inverter gate,' or orphan, of Poe's story, and it is just as easy to see that the concentric frames of paired elements create the nested marks of the calculus that leads to the connection of the innermost 'purloined' element with the outermost. This is the POV position, thanks to the 'blindness/invisibility' constructed in the middle. The invisible steals invisibility (the letter) in a moment constructed so that the Other will be blind, S(A̸).

It would be interesting to pursue this idea of 'optical sorites' in greater detail with Lacan's essay at hand. I am interested in how sorites models the process of gradual capture of the presubjective human, in traps preset by the Symbolic, to produce a 'hysterical subject' in relation to the blindness/lack of the Other.[32] Clearly, Diego Velázquez's 'meta-painting,' *Las Meninas* (1656), and Hans Holbein's *The Ambassadors* (1533) just as clearly develop optical traps within highly structured protocols that combine visibility and invisibility within tight 'autoerotic' circuits. Films, particularly those involving the device of the death dream (e.g., *Mulholland Drive*, *The Wizard of Oz*, *Vertigo*), engage autoeroticism at the level of identity and temporality. Equally, it would be interesting to reconsider Lacan's and Freud's camera analogies in light of the lens' theft of visibility (photographic capture) at the expense of 'freezing' the inhabitants of the view. The game of 'Blind Man's Bluff' displays just such a logic.

With such pop- and high-culture 'laboratories' providing new data and new perspectives, it would be useful to revisit Ellie Ragland's early work on the relation of Spencer-Brown's calculus to Lacan's topologies and deploy CDI in relation to the death drive, autoeroticism, and hysteria—and then review their ethnographic functionalities afresh.

All these connections, it appears to me, depend on understanding the coincidence of distinction and indication onto-topologically and critically; all hinge on understanding how Spencer-Brown's Boolean algebra extends to *trans*-Boolean topologies that so closely coincide with Lacan's. Most of all, the triplicities of Lacan, Spencer-Brown Poe reveal the kinship of three thinkers, all three good at ciphers; they combine 'binary' investigations with an 'orthogonal' excursion into issues that link the unconscious with *automaton*. This, in itself, suggests that Freud's idea of the unconscious as a perfectly preserved subject-less 'trash pile' was not so far off the mark. Perhaps with this minor but necessary correction, even object-oriented ontologists will be persuaded to reevaluate the calculus to consider just how much Freudian–Lacanian psychoanalysis has to contribute to the project of objects without subjects.

Notes

1. Levi Bryant, 'Introduction: Towards a Finally Subjectless Object,' in *The Democracy of Objects* (Ann Arbor: Open Humanities Press, 2011). Online text accessed August 2016, http://www.oapen.org/view?docId=444377. Note that Bryant reverses Spencer-Brown's convention of designating innermost spaces as unmarked and external graphic grounds as marked, suggesting that he considers being contained equivalent to being marked. Spencer-Brown's calculus is a favorite reference for other scholars working in this area, such as sociologist Niklas Luhmann, autopoieticists Francisco Varela and Humberto Maturano, and architectural theorist Patrik Schumacher. For an overview of extensions of Spencer-Brown's calculus, see Michael Schiltz, 'Space Is the Place: The Laws of Form and Social Systems,' *Thesis Eleven* 88 (February 2007): 8–30.
2. Bryant, 'The Closure of Objects,' 4.1, in op. cit: 'Spencer-Brown's point is any indication requires a distinction if the indication is to be made.... Form is the condition under which indication is possible.'
3. George Spencer-Brown, *Laws of Form* (London: Allen and Unwin, 1969), p. 1. I have benefited greatly from Ellie Ragland's pioneering study of Spencer-Brown's Lacanian connections in 'Lacan's Topological Unit and the Structure of Mind,' in *Lacan: Topologically Speaking*, ed. Ellie Ragland and Dragan Milovanovic (New York: Other Press, 2004), pp. 49–72. Ragland was the first Lacanian, I believe, to stress the coincidence of distinction and indication. (Ragland uses 'indiction' for 'indication,' which has the supplementary sense of a decree or declaration). I wish also to thank Todd McGowan, Alireza Moharar, and my editors, Jonathan Michael Dickstein and Gautam Basu Thakur for their helpful reviews of this chapter and its ideas in its various stages.
4. Louis Kauffman, 'Laws of Form: An Exploration in Mathematics and Foundations,' Rough Draft, 2014. Online text accessed Aug 2016,

http://homepages.math.uic.edu/~kauffman/Laws.pdf; hereinafter cited as 'Exploration.'

5. Pierre Skriabine, 'Clinic and Topology: The Flaw in the Universe,' in Ragland and Milovanovic, op. cit., p. 88.
6. Ellie Ragland, 'Lacan's Topological Unit and the Structure of Mind,' in Ragland and Milovanovic, op. cit., p. 54. Ragland quotes Lacan in Seminar XX (1972–1973), pp. 118–119.
7. George Spencer-Brown, *Laws of Form*, Limited Edition (Portland, OR: Cognizer Co., 1994), p. vii.
8. Louis Armand comments on Lacan's need for non-Boolean logic in 'Symptom in the Machine: Lacan, Joyce, Sollers,' 2007. Online text accessed Aug 2016, http://www.lacan.com/sympmach.htm
9. Ibid.
10. Ibid.
11. James Joyce, *Finnegans Wake*, Viking Compass Edition (New York: The Viking Press, 1967), p. 185.
12. Spencer-Brown (1994), p. 76.
13. Robert Samuels, 'Logical Time and *Jouissance*,' *Newsletter of the Freudian Field* 4, 1/2 (Spring/Fall 1990): 69–77; Jacques Lacan (1945), 'Logical Time and the Assertion of Anticipated Certainty,' in *Écrits*, trans. Bruce Fink (New York: W. W. Norton., 2002), pp. 161–175.
14. Bruce Fink, *The Lacanian Subject: Between Language and Jouissance* (Princeton: Princeton University, 1995), p. 14ff. Analyzing Lacan's use of ciphering to describe the unconscious, Fink makes this astounding claim on page 22: '…[T]his way of conceptualizing the unconscious [as an *automaton*] apparently leaves *no room for a subject of any kind.* …[T]here is absolutely no need to postulate any kind of consciousness of this automatic movement…[which] contains "indelible knowledge" which at the same time is "absolutely not subjectivized"' (Seminar XXI, February 12, 1974). Any objective reader of the texts of speculative realists would have to wonder, is this not precisely what they have been looking for?
15. Louis Kauffman details the ways the calculus connects to the primary algebra of $x^2 + ax + b = 0$, a recursive condition that leads to the 'Hegelian' paradox, J = ~J. 'Knot Logic and Topological Quantum Computing with Majorana Fermions,' in *Quantum Physics* (Ithaca: Cornell University Library, January 2013). Online text accessed Feb 2017, https://arxiv.org/abs/1301.6214

16. Louis Kauffman's interest in the form's inherent capability of reentering itself is summarized in the idea of the eigenform: 'What is an eigenform? An eigenform is a solution to an equation, a solution that occurs at the level of form, not at the level of number. You live in a world of eigenforms. You thought that those forms you see are actually "out there"? Out where? It has to be asked. The very space, the context that you regard as your external world is an eigenform. It is your organism's solution to the problem of distinguishing itself in a world of actions.' Kauffman seems to provide Lacan with the mathematical basis for his rejection, on the behalf of triplicity, of the need for 'pictorial' ideas of settings, contexts, and temporalities. Kauffman (2014), op. cit.
17. Ragland and Milovanovic (2004), p. 53. I would invoke Heraclitus on this matter. Beyond *palintropos harmoniē* of contradictory elements, Spencer-Brown's and Kauffman's idea of *Eigenform* suggests the Heraclitan alternative, *palintonos harmoniē,* a 'musical' and 'architectural' joint to replace the alternating current of contradiction. See this in Plato's revised terms, in Kelsey Wood, *Troubling Play: Meaning and Entity in Plato's Parmenides* (Albany: SUNY Press, 2005).
18. I borrow Lucretius's word for turbulence with an eye to other Latin terms in Harold Bloom's description of poetic anxiety: *askesis*, *tesseræ*, *dæmon*, *apophrades*, and *kenosis*. The metalepsis of creating something from nothing—'form' as Spencer-Brown would refer to it—requires all six, but we might focus first on *dæmon*, the most mechanical and nonhuman of the set. Harold Bloom, *The Anxiety of Influence: A Theory of Poetry* (Oxford: Oxford University Press, 1997).
19. Jacques Lacan, Seminar on 'The Purloined Letter,' in *Écrits: The First Complete Edition in English*, trans. Bruce Fink (New York: W. W. Norton, 2002), p. 17.
20. Edgar Allan Poe, 'The Purloined Letter,' in *The Complete Tales and Poems of Edgar Allan Poe* (New York: Vintage, 1975), p. 217.
21. Lacan (2002), p. 20.
22. The double channel idea is the basis of the phenomenon of 'cross-inscription,' a fundamental counterpart to relations of extimity (*extimité*). For example, in Ernst Jentsch's binary of the uncanny, 'the living person haunted by the specter of death' and 'the dead person carried by momentum past the instant of literal dying,' we say that death is inscribed into life just as life is inscribed into death, in effect that life/death are cross-inscribed binaries that, in 'ethnographic conditions' are

experienced in one of two ways. Ernst Jentsch, 'Zur Psychologie des Unheimlichen,' *Psychiatrisch-Neurologische Wochenschrift* 8, 22 (26 Aug): 195–198; 8, 23 (1 Sept): 203–205, 1906.

23. Kauffman, 'Exploration' (2014). Lacanians will easily see how the converter gate represents the function of *jouissance* in its ability to 'create value' out of either a negative or positive circuit flow. The single-gate circuit is thus Spencer-Brown's counterpart to the gapped circle of the death drive, where repetition compulsion creates a closed system that mimics the energetics of megalomania in its delusional relations to objects with demonic capabilities (Eros).
24. Lacan (2002), p. 10.
25. To understand the clever relationship between the constructed *poché* of pickpockets and S(Ⱥ), see Adam Greene, 'Profiles: Apollo Robbins,' *The New Yorker Magazine* (7 Jan 2013). Online text accessed Nov 2016, http://www.newyorker.com/magazine/2013/01/07/a-pickpockets-tale
26. Poe's description of the poet as being 'at one *remove* from a fool' [emphasis mine] sets up the idea of a poetry *with* mathematics in a very Spencer-Brownian fashion, especially because Dupin, in stealing the letter, is also fooling the *mathematical-poetical* Minister by 're-entering the form.'
27. For the tradition of Hermes' secrets, see Norman O. Brown, *Hermes the Thief: The Evolution of a Myth* (Madison: University of Wisconsin, 1947); and Leonard Barkan, 'Diana and Actæon: The Myth as Synthesis,' *English Literary Renaissance* 10, 3 (Sept): 317–359, 1980. Hermes' thievery equates with his ability to cross boundaries with impunity, including the arch-boundary separating death from life. Theft-by-stealth indicates that the binary involved with the concealment of the letter is not one of Bryant's 'flat binaries,' such as light/dark, but rather an 'orthogonal' binary connecting the intimate (gaze) with the point of view.
28. Richard Kopley, *Edgar Allan Poe and the Dupin Mysteries* (New York: Palgrave/Macmillan, 2008), pp. 18–24.
29. One should note that the gaze and the acousmatic voice both involve 'predication reversal,' an extimacy that locates a subjective function at the kernel of the object. This back-flow of causality and signification invites one to look further into the way the calculus's inverter gate adjusts the 'check valve' uniflow of the Symbolic's causal and signifying chains.
30. Spencer-Brown (1994), pp. 123–35. Also see Lewis Carroll and William Warren Bartley, *Lewis Carroll's Symbolic Logic* (New York: C. N. Potter, 1977).

31. Slavoj Žižek, *The Most Sublime Hysteric: Hegel with Lacan*, trans. Thomas Scott-Railton (Cambridge, UK/Malden, MA: Polity Press, 2014), pp. 21–34.
32. I would follow and expand on Mladen Dolar's advice about the uncanny, that is it is not produced by the Enlightenment's banishment of religion (the standard view) but already present in the ethnographic evidence of rituals, folktales, superstitions, and prophylactic magic from shamanistic times onward. 'I Shall Be with You on Your Wedding-Night': Lacan and the Uncanny, *Rendering the Real* 58 (Autumn): 5–23, 1991.

Bibliography

Armand, Louis. 2007. Symptom in the Machine: Lacan, Joyce, Sollers. *Lacan Dot Com*. http://www.lacan.com/sympmach.htm. Accessed 5 Aug 2016.

Barkan, Leonard. 1980. Diana and Actæon: The Myth as Synthesis. *English Literary Renaissance* 10 (3): 317–59.

Bloom, Harold. 1997. *The Anxiety of Influence: A Theory of Poetry*. Oxford: Oxford University Press.

Brown, Norman O. 1947. *Hermes the Thief: The Evolution of a Myth*. Madison: University of Wisconsin Press.

Bryant, Levi. 2011. *The Democracy of Objects*. Ann Arbor: Open Humanities Press.

Dolar, Mladen. 1991. 'I Shall Be with You on Your Wedding-Night': Lacan and the Uncanny. *Rendering the Real* 58(Oct): 5–23.

Fink, Bruce. 1995. *The Lacanian Subject: Between Language and Jouissance*. Princeton: Princeton University Press.

Greene, Adam. 2013. Profiles: Apollo Robbins. *The New Yorker Magazine,* 7 Jan. http://www.newyorker.com/magazine/2013/01/07/a-pickpockets-tale. Accessed 18 Nov 2016.

Jentsch, Ernst. 1906. Zur Psychologie des Unheimlichen. *Psychiatrisch-Neurologische Wochenschrift* 8, 22 (26 Aug): 195–8; 8, 23 (1 Sept): 203–5.

Kauffman, Louis. 2013. Knot Logic and Topological Quantum Computing with Majorana Fermions. In *Quantum Physics*. Ithaca: Cornell University Library. https://arxiv.org/abs/1301.6214. Accessed 6 Feb 2017.

———. 2014. Laws of Form: An Exploration in Mathematics and Foundations, Rough Draft. http://homepages.math.uic.edu/~kauffman/Laws.pdf. Accessed 6 Aug 2016.

Kopley, Richard. 2008. *Edgar Allan Poe and the Dupin Mysteries*. New York: Palgrave Macmillan.
Lacan, Jacques. 2002. Seminar on 'The Purloined Letter.' In *Écrits: The First Complete Edition in English*, 6–48. Trans. Bruce Fink. New York: W. W. Norton.
Poe, Edgar Allan. 1975. The Purloined Letter. In *The Complete Tales and Poems of Edgar Allan Poe*, 208–22. New York: Vintage.
Ragland, Ellie, and Dragan Milovanovic, eds. 2004. *Lacan: Topologically Speaking*. New York: Other Press.
Samuels, Robert. 1990. Logical Time and Jouissance. *Newsletter of the Freudian Field* 4 (1/2): 69–77.
Schiltz, Michael. 2007. Space Is the Place: The Laws of Form and Social Systems. *Thesis Eleven* 88: 8–30.
Spencer-Brown, George. 1969. *Laws of Form*. London: Allen and Unwin.
Wood, Kelsey. 2005. *Troubling Play: Meaning and Entity in Plato's Parmenides*. Albany: SUNY Press.
Žižek, Slavoj. 2014. *The Most Sublime Hysteric: Hegel with Lacan*. Trans. Thomas Scott-Railton. Cambridge/Malden: Polity Press.

Like an Animal: A Simile Instead of a Subject

Todd McGowan

The Absolute Rupture

One of the simplest ways in which we have historically suggested the link between humans and other animals is by using animal terms to describe human behavior. Rather than describing someone's behavior through adjectives and adverbs that locate a behavior in relation to other human actions, we compare it to the actions of an animal. These kinds of comparisons take place all the time and function as a kind of descriptive shorthand. But this is not the full extent of their role.

The existence of animal metaphors in everyday parlance seems to testify overtly to our kinship with other animals. We can compare ourselves to animals because we are alike in various ways—or at least because we consider ourselves alike. Rather than revealing an otherwise obscured affiliation between human and animal, however, the animal terms used to describe human behavior paradoxically reveal our distinctiveness from

T. McGowan (✉)
University of Vermont, Burlington, VT, USA

G. Basu Thakur, J.M. Dickstein (eds.), *Lacan and the Nonhuman*,
The Palgrave Lacan Series, DOI 10.1007/978-3-319-63817-1_9

the animal world. We do not describe the everyday or typical actions of humans in animal terms but reserve these metaphors for the excess of our subjectivity, a tendency that reveals what is at work in such descriptions. Animal metaphors are popular because they enable one to disavow the trauma of subjectivity's excess by naturalizing it.

The use of the animal metaphor articulates in a disguised form the violence of an absolute break between subjectivity and animality. Subjectivity is the struggle with this break, with an inability to be just another animal. Throughout history, subjects have concocted mechanisms for addressing the trauma of the break (such as seeing it as divinely instituted), but now the situation is dramatically different. The break has become increasingly less self-evident. The distinction between human and animal has come under fire from many quarters during preceding decades. Animal rights activists, materialist philosophers, deconstructionists, and especially evolutionary scientists have all called this absolute distinction into question. It is clear that other animals evince many of the characteristics once thought to be monopolized by humanity—communication, compassion, and even advanced thinking. The difference in kind has become a difference in degree in the aftermath of the Darwinian Revolution.

Initially, the Darwinian Revolution disturbed human exceptionalism, provoking vehement attacks bent on defending the elevation of the human above animality. These attacks continue even to the present day among fundamentalists who reject evolution in favor of creationism.[1] Although proponents of creationism occasionally achieve ideological victories, their position has become a minority one, especially among the educated populace. In the contemporary world, the animality of the human has become commonsensical.

This is why explanations about human behavior often focus on analogues among other animals. For instance, a male's aggressive dominance calls to mind the behavior of the alpha chimp, while the pick-up artist's fancy attire evinces peacocking. Most accept without question that many types of behavior that stand out in society have their roots in what humans share with animals. These explanations seem so convincing to contemporary ears because we have accepted that the human has not broken from its animality.

In one sense, there is no doubt that the human is an animal. Nevertheless, it is also clear that the emergence of subjectivity causes human animality to undergo a radical transformation. A rupture occurs when the human animal acquires the ability to speak and thus to become a subject. The speaking subject is no longer directly an animal but must relate to its animality indirectly. It is not simply ideology or human narcissism that has led to the insistence on the subject's exceptionality.[2] The exceptional status of the speaking subject in relation to the animal world constantly confronts one when witnessing subjects acting in ways that animals do not. It is not that subjects can surpass animals in their intellectual achievements or cultural accomplishments but that they indulge in excesses that one cannot find in the animal world.

This is the fundamental problem with the theorization of the distinction between humans and animals put forward by Aristotle. For Aristotle, reason separates the human soul from the animal. The human has the capacity to follow the guidance of its rationality when it acts, whereas the animal is the slave of its passions and appetites.[3] Even though this version of the distinction between humans and animals has predominated for centuries, it completely fails to account for the ability of some animals to act with rational calculation, and more important, for the distinctively human acts that have nothing to do with rational calculation—religious fanaticism, skydiving, overeating, and so on.

Immanuel Kant gives the distinction a much more tenable foundation. Kant recognizes the ability of the subject to give itself a law as the source of the break from natural being. As he formulates it, the subject paradoxically proves its freedom only through the assertion of a law that demands obedience. The law that the subject asserts, however, creates room for disobedience. Although laws govern the natural world, they differ in kind from the laws that subjects give to themselves because they cannot be disobeyed. Obeying the law of gravity is not the same as obeying the speed limit, even though natural law theorists attempt to put them on the same level.[4] Rocks cannot decide not to fall, whereas subjects are able to not drive too fast.

After Kant, it becomes clear that the law, not rationality as such, separates the subject from its own animality.[5] Even if it would like to, the subject of law cannot act in an immediately natural way. It relates to its natural being through the mediation of law that deracinates it from this being. For the subject of law, to act naturally is to unnaturally act naturally. A basic alienation characterizes the individual that has been subjected to the law.

The uprooting that law enacts does not produce a subject harmoniously integrated into the social order. Instead, it produces a subject excessively attached to the law and its prohibition. The law commands a renunciation, but this renunciation itself produces its own form of enjoyment—what Jacques Lacan calls surplus enjoyment. As Lacan puts it in his *Seminar XVI*: 'Surplus enjoyment is a function of the renunciation of enjoyment under the effect of discourse.'[6] In the act of barring enjoyment to the speaking subject, the law creates an excess that haunts the subject. This occurs because the enjoyment that the law demands the subject renounce does not exist prior to its renunciation. In effect, the subject renounces an enjoyment into existence through the prohibition that the law lays down.

The most conspicuous excesses of subjectivity (for instance, orgies, drug overdoses, killing sprees) are not the most common. The excess of subjectivity entails primarily an obscene attachment to the law itself. This attachment stems from the exclusive role that the law plays in producing the subject's capacity to enjoy itself. Thanks to the law, one can enjoy activities that otherwise would not be pleasurable such as doing one's job or preparing dinner or even engaging in strenuous exercise. The subject's attachment to the law is unconscious but has the effect of transforming everything that she or he does into a site of enjoyment.

Even extreme activities provide the enjoyment that they do through the law that mediates them. Participation in orgies always occurs against the backdrop of a law that enjoins them, and it is this backdrop that provides enjoyment for the subject. The serial killer finds enjoyment in killing because it violates the law, even though no serial killers consciously avow the part that the law plays in their murders. Serial killing is unthinkable without the primacy of the law. But the primary enjoyment that the law creates occurs in obedience to it. Subjects excessively attach themselves to the law so that they derive enjoyment from obeying it. Subjects of the law cannot obey neutrally but do so through a passionate investment in the constraint that the law imposes.[7]

Law distorts the way that the subject performs even the most natural activities (such as eating, sleeping, having sex, and working). Each of these activities ceases to serve the subject's survival and becomes a possible end in itself because of the intervention of law, which restricts how much the subject can eat, sleep, or have sex, while compelling it to work. Insomnia is just one indicator of the impact of the law on a seemingly natural activity. Law penetrates all aspects of subjectivity.

The law does not play this structuring role for other animals.[8] They avoid the obscene attachment to the law that plagues speaking subjects. Animals may kill, grieve, feel pleasure, or display compassion, but the excess of the law invades only the speaking subject. For this reason, comparison to animals holds a great appeal for subjects. They resort to animal metaphors to convince themselves that the result of their obscene attachment to the law is simply a natural phenomenon and has nothing obscene about it.

The animal metaphor is an act of disavowal. Rather than disavowing animality (as one might expect), we disavow the obscene excess that accompanies subjectivity and that renders us unnatural beings. We do not experience shame for the animal that remains in us but for the excess of subjectivity that the image of animality hides.[9] The disavowal that occurs in the animal metaphor enables us simultaneously to recognize this obscene excess and to attribute it to an animality for which we are not responsible. Through the animal metaphor, humiliating excesses become the result of a natural inheritance imposed on us and have nothing to do with how we organize our enjoyment.

The Strained Simile

Some of the most hackneyed similes in the English language concern animality. Most animal similes have become so overused that we not only avoid them in written work but even in casual conversation, except insofar as we employ these similes with ironic distance. Very few people recite similes such as 'hungry like a wolf,' 'sneaky as a snake,' 'sly as a fox,' 'busy as a beaver,' 'wise as an owl,' or 'stubborn as a mule.' These are no longer active similes but have become clichés. At the same time, the commonsensical status of these similes sheds light on how the use of animality in reference to speaking subjects' functions.

The similes that refer to animals do so in order to point out a subject acting outside the norms that typically govern subjectivity. Rather than eating calmly, someone eats as if he is as hungry as a wolf. Rather than saying the expected, someone else gives a response that shows she is as wise as an owl. What stands out about these animal similes is how little they typically have to do with the animals to which they refer. Wolves are not necessarily hungrier than other animals, and nothing in the comportment of owls displays unusual wisdom. Occasionally, one of the similes does hit the mark: the ox really does possess extraordinary strength, although even in this case there are better candidates (like the elephant or the gorilla) for the simile.[10]

The existence of inaccurate similes is not just the result of limited human knowledge of how animals actually act—no one verified the relative voraciousness of the wolf before creating the simile—but also follows from the function of the animal simile itself. The inaccurate simile is the paradigmatic case, whereas the accurate one is the exception that hides the function of the simile. The accuracy of the simile ultimately is contingent because the point is not to accurately account for a human activity with an animal comparison but instead to naturalize this activity. In this sense, it does not matter which animal we align with the activity as long as there is an animal that serves to represent it.

Animal similes have a dual function. On the one hand, they express the excessiveness of the subject. We have recourse to an animal comparison when an action goes beyond the bounds of everyday human life, and we imagine that the animal embodies this particular excess. On the other hand, however, we use the comparison in order to characterize the specific excess as natural rather than as an effect of subjectivity itself. Lacking the law of the signifier, animals, even though they can be extreme, cannot be excessive.

A look at body fat reveals this point. We live during a contemporary obesity epidemic in which a large percentage of the population eats excessively. According to standard measures of obesity, most whales throughout the history of their species would be obese. Whales can have 50% body fat—in this sense, 'fat as a whale' is an accurate simile—but they cannot suffer from obesity. That is to say, whales cannot transform eating into the single act that gives significance to their existence in the way that the speaking subject can. Whales undoubtedly find pleasure in eating, but they cannot enjoy it.[11] They cannot eat too excess in order to transgress a social restriction that commands a healthy body.

A vast quantity of fat serves a necessary function for whales that it does not serve for subjects.[12] Nonetheless, even though whales are fat, subjects have the capacity to be fatter. Given the subject's capacity for enjoying the restriction that it violates, it is not surprising that the fattest subject easily surpasses the fattest whale in terms of percentage of body fat. The advantage that subjects have lies in their ability to sublimate—to derive all their satisfaction from an otherwise mundane process. The subject cannot simply eat like other animals but must relate to eating through the law. The more that the law restricts how much one should eat, the more enjoyment one locates in the act of eating.[13] As a result, obesity epidemics are possible among speaking subjects in a way that they are not among whales, an inherently fatter species than humans.

Identifying this excess with the law indicates the fundamental disharmony that defines subjectivity, which is why we disavow its relationship to subjectivity through the animal simile. When one says that a friend is as 'fat as a whale,' one not only articulates this friend's excessiveness but also divorces the excess from subjectivity. By associating fatness with a whale rather than with the subject, the insult, in addition to wounding the friend's psyche, has the effect of naturalizing the unnatural act of eating too much.

Animal similes function to hide the unnatural entity—that is, the subject in its excessiveness—that the mediation of the signifier produces. The animal simile enables us to imagine ourselves as natural beings and thereby to domesticate the trauma of the excess of subjectivity to which we apply the parallel. We have recourse to animal descriptions of our activity precisely when that activity most violently separates us from the natural world.

We describe subjects in animal terms not when they act in ordinary ways but when they commit heinous acts of aggression, when they indulge in licentious sexuality, or when they enjoy themselves beyond the bounds of propriety. Someone attacks a victim like a 'mad dog'; another has sex like an 'animal'; and someone else laughs like a 'hyena.' In each of these cases, the use of an animal simile designates an excess linked to a particular animal or to animality in general. But what stands out from these comparisons is their inappropriateness.

Speaking subjects are capable of more aggression than the most rabid dog: No dog managed to kill 100,000 people with a single gesture like the pilot of the plane who dropped the atomic bomb on Hiroshima, and no dog has ever perpetuated a mass shooting at an elementary school. The idea is absurd. Likewise, animals have never approached the sexual creativity of subjects, nor has the hyena created an entire artistic genre devoted to producing laughter. Animal sexuality is shockingly mundane when compared to its human counterpart. When people think of themselves as having sex animalistically, they never are. The wild sex act is the unique province of speaking subjects. The animal similes that we use never come close to hitting the mark, and yet we persist in using them.

As subjects, we always relate excessively to the world. We do not simply eat but enjoy the prospect of eating too much. We do not simply have sex but invent perverse rituals to render the sexual act more satisfying. Even our everyday relationship to the world bears the marks of excess. Subjectivity signals our inability to relate directly to the objects around us or even to ourselves. The speaking subject can never simply see what it sees or hear what it hears. Instead, it sees and hears through the distortion of the signifier, a distortion that forecloses any direct contact with the world.

Stuck in a position of alienation from the world, we use animal terms to describe ourselves in order to take up the direct relation to the world we imagine that animals have. The animal has an imaginary immediacy that subjects believe themselves to have lost, and the animal simile is an effort to recapture this lost immediacy, which we never actually had.[14] The necessity of indirection—the fact of mediation—is what the animal simile attempts to spare us from. We place our excessive relation to the world in animal terms in order simultaneously to indicate and obscure its excessiveness. This is at work even when animal terms seem most like the appropriate expression to communicate the subject's activity.

For What Are We Rooting?

Of all the nicknames used to identify American sports teams, animal names compose a solid plurality. In the National Football League, where this phenomenon is most pronounced, 14 of the 32 teams have animal nicknames.[15] In the National Basketball Association, in Major League Baseball, and in the National Hockey League, the number is 8 out of 30. The other nicknames are a mélange of various occupations (e.g., Packers, Steelers, Brewers), exotic characters (e.g., Wizards, Pirates, Angels), geographical features (e.g., Lakers, Avalanche, Rockies), meteorological phenomena (e.g., Heat, Thunder, Hurricanes), or racist appellations (e.g., Redskins, Chiefs, Blackhawks). Each of these other types of team nickname connotes excess, whether it is above normal temperatures, supernatural powers, or just heightened production of a certain commodity. In each sport, however, it is animal nicknames that always outnumber all other types. Even more than Buccaneers or Saints, animals serve as figures of excess for players and fans, and they provide a point of identification through this excess.

Sport is an arena of excess. Athletes spend time training for their sports that they might use preparing for activities that would benefit society (like going to medical school) or secure their own future (like studying to become an investment banker). Although a few top athletes reap a financial windfall from playing their sports, most do not, and time invested in sports training, if the ultimate goal is a monetary reward or benefitting society, is largely wasted time.

But the lack of utility associated with sports is extrinsic to the satisfaction that sports provide. No one buys tickets to watch brain surgeons operate or investment bankers compete against each other. The utility of these activities militates against the possibility that they could play the role that sports play in contemporary society. The absence of any utility in sport is a condition of possibility for spectators to enjoy it.[16] Sport is an excessive enterprise, one that uses up an incredible quantity of both individual and social resources without returning any tangible utility for either the individual or the society.

The excesses of sport become clearly visible in all the rituals that surround the games. Otherwise sensible adults dress up in costumes, paint their faces, dye their hair, and spend thousands of dollars all to display their allegiance to a particular team that does not reciprocate the intensity of the feeling. Sports' fandom is a distinctly lopsided love affair: The true fan would never simply decide to root for a new team, whereas from the team's perspective, one fan is as good as another. They are replaceable entities for the team to which they grant a sublime importance. There is thus something shameful about being a fan. One devotes oneself excessively to a team that displays no devotion in return.

As a fan, one is always on the verge of total humiliation because of this one-sided devotion. Looking at what fans do without the lens of sublimation renders everything completely ridiculous—the costumes, the painted faces, the dyed hair, the wasted money. Fans avoid seeing their behavior in this way by committing themselves fully to their investment. The excessiveness of the commitment, however, cannot but draw attention to itself. Sports' fandom reveals the trauma of the subject's excessive attachment more than any other realm.

Given the excessive nature of sport, it is not surprising that so many team names involve animals. The animal name expresses this excess by indicating that everything associated with sport transcends the everyday human realm. The problem is that the source of the subjects' excessiveness is not its animality but its subjectivity. In this sense, the proper name of every sports team should be the Subjects, despite the repetitiveness. Sport is the exclusive province of the speaking subject. Its excessiveness has no animal parallel.

Nonetheless, we resort the animal nicknames for teams in order to transform sport into play, to naturalize the unnatural activity. Although animals of all stripes spend time playing, none invest themselves in sport the way in which speaking subjects do. Sport is not just an extension of play, a human version of animal play. A lack of seriousness defines play: While at play, animals and humans engage in activities that could be serious without treating them seriously. A cat playing at trying to seize a piece of string from its human partner does not really want to have the string but merely wants to play at having it. Two dogs playing with each other act as if they are fighting but do not try to injure the other. While just playing, humans hit the tennis ball to each other without starting a game or keeping score. These cases all exemplify play rather than sport.

Play becomes sport at the moment it becomes serious. Sport is play taken seriously—for example, when a tennis match begins after two friends stop just hitting the ball back and forth. A radical break occurs between the act of hitting a tennis ball and the commencement of a tennis match. Although one can invest oneself in the activity of play, sport engenders an excessive investment because of its seriousness. Often, the result of a sporting event can matter more to spectators than the fate of their relationships or their physical health. We can see heroism in a player participating in the Super Bowl with a broken leg because we understand the grave seriousness of the activity. It is not just a game. Sport can create significance, which definitely separates it from play. Nonetheless, sports fans avoid confronting the fact of this excessiveness.

The naturalization of sport enables subjects to disavow their excessive investment in an inherently insignificant activity. More than any other activity, sport is the site for sublimation: Individuals give outsized importance to an activity that has nothing to do with human survival, self-interest, or sexual satisfaction. We resort to animal nicknames for sports teams so often because these names assist in the process of obscuring the obscenity (and thus the shame) of being a fan. But sport is a relatively benign realm, and the disavowal of our excess here seems harmless. The gravity of this disavowal becomes more apparent when we look at the role that animal metaphors play in our engagement with race.

The Racist Evasion

The explanation for the racist use of animal terms appears simple. By giving an animal description to someone of another race, the subject removes this other from the category of humanity, thereby licensing the same type of treatment that animals receive. If we can kill animals without repercussions, then we can do the same to the animalized other.[17] First, we debase the other, and then we are able to inflict all kinds of horrors on this person. For instance, in the act calling black people 'bucks' or 'coons,' the racist dehumanizes them by placing them on a lower evolutionary level. By doing so, one prepares the way for acts that fall outside human morality. According to this line of thought, it is a short step from this appellation to lynching the black individual just as one would hunt and kill a male deer or a raccoon. The metaphor, even when it remains unarticulated, makes inhuman violence possible.

In his analysis of the Nazi Final Solution, Giorgio Agamben sees exactly this operation at work. Jews became the lowest form of animal life, which served as a necessary prelude to their extinction. In *Homo Sacer*, Agamben writes: 'The Jews were exterminated not in a mad and giant holocaust but exactly as Hitler had announced, "as lice," which is to say, as bare life. The dimension in which the extermination took place is neither religion nor law, but biopolitics.'[18] Agamben argues that the stripping away of the political being of the Jews and their reduction to bare animal life was propaedeutic to the extermination. The reduction to animality enabled Nazi soldiers to enact the annihilation as if they were fumigating Germany.

Even the most committed vegans have no second thoughts about delousing their hair when lice infest it. If animal metaphors convinced Nazis that Jews were nothing more than lice, this eliminated any moral compunction that they might have had about perpetuating the Final Solution. It is difficult to kill human beings, but not lice. Hitler's own words seem to suggest the nefarious power of the animal metaphor and its role in the extermination of the Jews.

The Holocaust, like lynching in the United States, appears to function as an absolute proof of the dangerous endpoint of animal metaphors. Who could deny the direct line from the animal metaphor to the death camps? But precisely when we think of it in these terms, the logic of the homology in the simple explanation breaks down completely. The way that Nazis and white racists perpetuated their crimes gives the lie to the attempt to connect these crimes to the animalization of their victims. These crimes betray an excess that does not typically occur in the treatment of animals.

Despite Hitler's claim, the Nazis did not exterminate the Jews like lice but actually treated them far worse than an exterminator would treat lice. No louse ever had to file before an anonymous judge that would contingently decide whether it lived or died. No louse was ever forced to participate in the act of its own extermination. Before being killed, Jews endured humiliation and constant debasement. What's more, after their deaths, the Nazis burned their bodies so that there would be no trace left of them. Nazis did not target Jews as animals but as excessive subjects whose excess represented an existential threat to the German nation. In comparison, lice being exterminated get off easy.

This dynamic is even more evident in the violence of lynching. We might think that the term 'buck' prepares the way for the lynching of black men. But no one has ever lynched a male deer, and perpetuators of lynching do not typically eat the victim as they do when they kill a deer. Hunters do not burn deer alive. It also probably is safe to say that no one who has hunted a deer in the history of humanity has stuffed the deer's testicles in the animal's mouth prior to killing it, though doing this to a black man was a relatively common practice among those who lynched.

In short, we do not treat the targets of racism in the same way that we treat animals, even though we use animal terms to describe the former. This difference in treatment suggests that the animal metaphor is not functioning to animalize the people to whom one applies it. The aim of the animal term cannot be to position the so-named people so that they can then be treated like animals because we use the animal term to treat people in ways that we would never treat the animals. There must be another operation at work.

If we examine how the racist term 'buck' functions, it is evident that it has nothing to do with animality, although it enables the subject employing it to imagine just such an association. Actual bucks do not display the excessive sexuality that the appellation connotes. They are no more sexually driven than males of other animal species. The term 'buck' does not indicate a link between the sexuality of the black man and that of a male deer, but it registers the racist fantasy of a black sexuality that surpasses the merely human sexuality of whites. Rather than being less than human, the figure of the buck is a figure of superhuman (or supermasculine) sexuality.

This fantasy of black sexuality plays a pivotal role in the sexual enjoyment of the racist subject, who enjoys through the fantasy of excessive black enjoyment. This image of excess creates a path for the racist subject's own enjoyment, which occurs in the form of identification with the black other. Of course, no one could avow this enjoyment because it exposes the parasitic relationship that the racist subject has with black sexuality. No racists can admit that their own sexual enjoyment depends on that of the black other. The animal metaphor of the buck enables racist subjects to disavow the source of their own enjoyment.

There is an implicit theory of sexual enjoyment that resides in the association of the racialized other with animal sexuality. If black sexuality is excessive and at the same time natural, there is no mediation to impair its excessiveness. Even though the animal metaphor is demeaning, it also strips the black subject of the lack that accompanies subjectivity. A pure sexuality emerges out of this metaphor. Using the term 'buck' enables speaking subjects to imagine that their sexuality allows a complete enjoyment not denatured through the defiles of lack.

Even when the racist animal metaphor is not sexual, it nonetheless always concerns the other's enjoyment and an attempt to link that enjoyment to the natural world. If we examine the other racist animal term for blackness, 'coon,' we find no sexual connotations but nevertheless a clear link to enjoyment. The image of the 'coon' indicates easy laughter and excessive amusement. Although the term derives from the raccoon, the associations that accompany it have little to do with the behavior of actual raccoons, who do not seem especially jovial in comparison with the rest of the animal world. Even more than is the case with the figure of the buck, here the animal metaphor evinces distance from animality.

Racism always involves denigration. This is why it seems as if the racist use of animal terms aims at placing the racialized other outside humanity and on the same plane of other animals. This is undoubtedly the conscious intention of the person who employs animal metaphors as racial slurs. The slurs, however, state the opposite of what the speaker consciously intends. The animal metaphor indicates a point at which the racialized other fails to act like an animal, and it is this transcendence of animality that the racist subject both finds traumatic and enjoys. What bothers and thrills the subject in the racialized other is not the proximity of the other to animality but the excess of subjectivity and thus the enjoyment that the other evinces. The animal metaphor enables the subject to access the other's enjoyment while obscuring its excessiveness.

'The Beast with Two Backs'

The mismatch between actual animal activity and the human act named by an animal metaphor becomes most acute in the famous opening scene from *Othello*, when Iago and Roderigo awaken Brabantio in the middle of the night to tell him that Othello and Desdemona have eloped. On three occasions when he calls out to Brabantio, Iago employs animal metaphors to describe the sexual activity of Othello and Desdemona. He uses these terms to horrify the white father by appealing to his racism. But the way that Shakespeare deploys the series of images has the effect of revealing the hidden truth of the animal description—that it has nothing at all to do with animality.

Iago's first statement highlights the immediacy of the sexual act taking place between Othello and Desdemona; he exclaims: 'Even now, now, very now, an old black ram/Is tupping your white ewe.'[19] The vision of Othello as a lascivious black animal obviously plays on traditional racist ideas, but Iago's metaphor transforms Desdemona into an animal as well, albeit an innocent one. It is this transformation that stands out because it simultaneously connotes excessive sexuality and a natural act. Iago expresses excess through recourse to nature.

Soon after this initial metaphor, Iago follows up by describing the potential result of the sexual liaison in animal terms. He says to Brabantio: '[Y]ou'll/have your daughter covered with a Barbary horse,/you'll have your nephews neigh to you.'[20] Here, Iago resorts to a different animal metaphor and uses it to convince Brabantio of the imminent threat that animality poses to him, that he is on the verge of being related to animals. It seems as if we should take Iago at his word and conclude that what really horrifies us is the idea of our animality. Nonetheless, this would miss what the idea of animality conveys. Iago does not describe Othello in animal terms because he acts like an animal but because he does not.

It is Othello's failure to act like an animal—his ability to speak poetically—that neither Iago nor Brabantio can countenance. Othello's excess has a clear attachment to signification rather than natural sexuality. Even though he is a warrior, in the first scene in which he appears Othello uses poetry to avoid a fight. When Desdemona's father and his men threaten Othello, he responds: 'Keep up your bright swords, for the dew will rust them./Good signior, you shall command more with years/Than with your weapons.'[21] Here, Othello reveals his ability to act with words, which is the unique province of subjectivity.

It also is clear that Othello's poetic rendering of his heroism provides the key to successfully wooing Desdemona. Rather than seducing her with his raw sexuality (as Iago's metaphors suggest), Othello relies exclusively on his poetry. He is perhaps the greatest poet that Shakespeare created.[22] This excess within language disturbs Iago and Brabantio precisely because it is not profoundly Other, not part of a natural animality that they have left behind. It is the excess of Othello's subjectivity itself, and Iago's metaphors attempt to mask Othello's subjectivity in the guise of animality.

Iago's final use of an animal metaphor to describe Othello and Desdemona represents a departure from the first two. Whereas the earlier metaphors ensconce themselves entirely within the animal world, the third suggests that the real trauma of the liaison does not reside in its animality. When Brabantio asks Iago to identify himself, rather than answer, Iago states: 'I am one, sir, that comes to tell you your daughter/ and the Moor are now making the beast with two backs.'[23] Iago's metaphor, which is Shakespeare's own invention and has no known precedent, aims at continuing to shock Brabantio by repeating the image of his daughter returned to an animal state in the thrall of a black man.

Like the earlier metaphors Iago employs, this one plays on the association of the blackness of the Moor with animality; however, what stands out about it is the mismatch between the metaphor and the animal version of the act it recounts. Even though Iago describes the sexual encounter between Othello and Desdemona as a 'beast with two backs,' this image does not accurately represent most animal copulation. Humans do not have a monopoly on face-to-face sex, but it is extremely rare in the animal world. Certainly no animals that Iago would have seen engaged in it.[24] To describe an activity that separates speaking subjects from their animal relatives using animal terms indicates that it is not simply a question of debasing Othello. It is also a way of transforming the excessive form of the subject's sexuality into a natural act.

Through the progression of insults that Shakespeare has Iago use to describe Othello, he lays bare the underlying logic of racist animal imagery as such. Subjects turn to animal terms to express pejorative sentiments in order to create a natural way of being that does not exist. The association of racial otherness with nature enables the subject to disavow not its own naturalness but its lack in the racial other. The animal metaphor debases the racialized other and simultaneously preserves the image of this other as a natural whole able to enjoy itself directly without the mediating constraints of the signifier. The fantasy of an unalloyed natural being lurks within every animal insult. This enables the insulting subject to sustain the image of complete enjoyment not mediated by law (and thus by lack) in the racialized other. The image of the other's complete enjoyment creates the illusory possibility of the subject's own.

The Absence of Natural Enjoyment

Animal metaphors can function as pleasant compliments or pave the way to genocide. Nevertheless, in either case, they enable subjects to disavow the excess of their subjectivity. The subject's excess is the origin of the trouble that it gives itself and the society in which it exists. Such excess manifests itself in the subject's inability to live out a harmonious existence, which leads the subject to avoid confronting the excess through whatever means it can find. The animal metaphor is the perfect form for the disavowal of excess because it attributes the excess to an animality that itself has no subjectivity. Once the excess appears natural, it ceases to be excessive.

When we look empirically at animal metaphors, the lack of connection to actual animals does not seem apparent. The fact that subjects saw parallels between human behavior and that of other animals appears to be the self-evident source of these metaphors. Of course, there is some connection between the behavior of subjects and that of animals since subjects never escapes animality. But one must ask why these metaphors arise, especially in cases in which they do not correspond to any exceptional characteristic in the animal to which they refer.

The encounter with the excessiveness of subjectivity always traumatizes subjects. Whether it takes the form of a fraternity member drinking himself to death, a nun restraining from sexual activity throughout her life, an obsessional precisely arranging the utensils before every meal, or a child refusing to wear any color besides red, the excesses of subjectivity reveal that not only can the subject not exist in harmony with the social order but also that it cannot exist in harmony with itself. From this perspective, animals appear as harmonious beings.

If we could imagine ourselves as the kin of animals connected by the words 'like' or 'as,' we could eliminate our own obscene disharmony. We could avoid the traumatic shame that inheres in our subjectivity. The animal metaphor provides a clear path away from this shame. Nonetheless, the shame of subjectivity is also the site for the subject's freedom initiated by the law. To imagine oneself external to the shame of subjectivity in the cocoon of animal nature is to imagine oneself deprived of freedom.

Without the possibility of shame, freedom remains an impossibility. Shame stems from an unconscious recognition that there is no guarantee supporting one's existence. In the experience of shame, one confronts as defining absence where one expects to find an authority. As Joan Copjec puts it in *Imagine There's No Woman*: 'Shame is awakened not when one looks at oneself, or those whom one cherishes, through another's eyes, but when one suddenly perceives a lack in the Other.'[25] This perception of a lack in the Other that Copjec identifies with shame represents the moment when freedom becomes actual.

It is not coincidental that Jean-Paul Sartre, in his panegyric to freedom, *Being and Nothingness*, broaches the problem of shame. Freedom is inextricable from shame because both emerge simultaneously from the imposition of the law. Only a free Being can experience shame, which occurs at the moment when its dependence on the law becomes visible. This is what Sartre hints at when he contends that 'pure shame is…*recognizing myself* in this degraded, fixed, and dependent being which I am for the other.'[26] A subject experiences shame because the other sees the obscenity of dependence. Although a free subject, one has become attached to the law even—or especially—in the act of violating it.

Animal metaphors play a vital role in the disavowal of the excess that results from the human animal's subjection to the law. In response to this mass disavowal, however, we do not need to abandon the animal metaphor. We would not automatically grasp the excessiveness proper to subjectivity if we ceased to label someone 'fat as a whale.' The point instead is to know how to interpret such utterances. When we think we are comparing humans to animals, we are really attesting to the radicality of the distinction between them. We must hear the excess of subjectivity at the heart of the animal metaphor. We must see the freedom of the law in the subject eating like a horse.

Notes

1. See, for instance, Creation Minute at http://creationminute.com/
2. Freud characterizes Darwin's discovery of natural selection as one of the great wounds to human narcissism, along with the Copernican discovery of heliocentrism and his own discovery of the unconscious.
3. In the *Politics*, Aristotle formulates a homology between the distinction between human and animal on the one side, and man and woman or master and slave on the other. He claims: 'Whereas the lower animals cannot even apprehend reason; they obey their passions. And indeed the use made of slaves and of tame animals is not very different; for both with their body minister to the needs of life.' Aristotle, *Politics*, trans. B. Jowett, in *The Complete Works of Aristotle, Vol. 2*, ed. Jonathan Barnes (Princeton: Princeton University Press, 1984), pp. 1:5. Reason becomes the justification for all social hierarchies in Aristotle's political philosophy. The gift of reason frees men from occupying themselves with the needs of life and enables them to establish themselves as political beings.
4. This is the position developed most prominently by Thomas Aquinas. For Aquinas, there is no fundamental difference between laws of nature and moral laws because morality follows from humanity's rational nature.
5. Kant does call the subject's capacity to give itself a law the fact of reason, but it is reason in its practical use, not reason as the source of calculation.
6. Jacques Lacan, *Le Séminaire, Livre XVI: D'un Autre à l'Autre, 1968–1969*, ed. Jacques-Alain Miller (Paris: Seuil, 2006), p. 19.
7. Judith Butler theorizes the process of the subject attaching itself to the constraint of the law in *The Psychic Life of Power*, where she claims, 'there is no formation of the subject without a passionate attachment to subjection.' Judith Butler, *The Psychic Life of Power* (Stanford: Stanford University Press, 1997), p. 67.

8. Birds build nests to house their young but do not make the building of nests into an end in itself. In contrast, I can transform even an activity as banal as trading stocks into an end that I enjoy. As Hannah Arendt points out, work creates a world for subjects in a way that it does not for animals. See Hannah Arendt, *The Human Condition*, 2nd ed. (Chicago: University of Chicago Press, 1998).
9. Jean-Paul Sartre describes the experience of shame as that of being oneself in front of the other. The paradigmatic moment of shame is that of being caught spying through a keyhole. At this moment, the one who sees the subject illicitly looking exposes the excessive status of the subject's enjoyment.
10. The proper simile would be 'strong as a dung beetle,' given that this is likely the strongest animal on Earth relative to its size. Or, if one did not want to take size into account, the simile should be 'strong as an elephant.'
11. In contrast to pleasure, enjoyment requires the addition of some type of damage that the subject undergoes. There is no healthy enjoyment.
12. Evolutionary psychologists do explain the contemporary obesity epidemic by pointing out the role that fat storage had in human survival. A large quantity of body fat had a necessary function for humans. But subjectivity enables us to exceed the bounds of this necessity. No human being needed to eat itself into immobility to survive.
13. The anorexic's enjoyment of not eating also follows from the law's restriction of eating. This type of subject excessively attaches itself to the law's restriction. By obeying the law excessively, the anorexic actually disobeys it.
14. We do not know what mediation informs the relation to the world that animals have. As a result, the image of an immediate connection is only the product of the subject's fantasy.
15. The animal nicknames in the National Football League are: Atlanta Falcons, Arizona Cardinals, Baltimore Ravens, Carolina Panthers, Chicago Bears, Cincinnati Bengals, Denver Broncos, Detroit Lions, Indianapolis Colts, Jacksonville Jaguars, Los Angeles Rams, Miami Dolphins, Philadelphia Eagles, and Seattle Seahawks.
16. According to Kant, our ability to enjoy the beauty of an object depends on its lack of utility; he claims: 'Beauty is the form of the purposiveness of an object, insofar as it is perceived in it without representation of an end.' Immanuel Kant, *Critique of the Power of Judgment*, trans. Paul

Guyer and Eric Matthews (Cambridge: Cambridge University Press, 2000), p. 120. This is equally the case with sublime objects, which is where we should locate the sporting event.

17. This is the position of Charles Patterson in *Eternal Treblinka*. There, he states, 'with animals already defined as "lower life" fated for exploitation and slaughter, the designation of "lesser" humans as animals paved the way for their subjugation and destruction.' Charles Patterson, *Eternal Treblinka: Our Treatment of Animals and the Holocaust* (New York: Lantern Books, 2002), p. 26.
18. Giorgio Agamben, *Homo Sacer: Sovereign Power and Bare Life*, trans. Daniel Heller-Roazen (Stanford: Stanford University Press, 1998), p. 114.
19. William Shakespeare, *Othello*, in *The Riverside Shakespeare*, 2nd ed. (New York: Houghton Mifflin, 1996), I.i. pp. 97–98. Though there is considerable scholarly debate, it is at least likely that Othello and Desdemona never had time alone enough to have sex, at least after their marriage.
20. Ibid., I.i. pp. 124–126.
21. Ibid., I.ii. pp. 59–61.
22. This is a widely shared view, articulated most famously by renowned Shakespeare interpreter A. C. Bradley. Comparing Othello with Shakespeare's other heroes, Bradley writes, 'if one places side by side with these speeches an equal number by any other hero, one will not doubt that Othello is the greatest poet of them all.' A. C. Bradley, *Shakespearean Tragedy*, 2nd ed. (London: Macmillan, 1905), p. 188.
23. Shakespeare (1996), I.i. pp. 125–126.
24. Although other animals occasionally partake in face-to-face sex, it is only the bonobo that does so as a common practice.
25. Joan Copjec, *Imagine There's No Woman: Ethics and Sublimation* (Cambridge: MIT Press, 2002), p. 128.
26. Jean-Paul Sartre, *Being and Nothingness*, trans. Hazel E. Barnes (New York: Washington Square Press, 1956), p. 384. Sartre erroneously sees the dependence of the shamed subject on the other who sees it, when in fact it is the subject's dependence on the law that is the source of shame. Sartre misses this because his philosophy does not locate freedom in the imposition of the law, as Kant does. For Sartre, the subject is free based on its capacity for self-negation, though he never seeks the source of this capacity.

Bibliography

Agamben, Giorgio. 1998. *Homo Sacer: Sovereign Power and Bare Life*. Trans. Daniel Heller-Roazen. Stanford: Stanford University Press.

Arendt, Hannah. 1998. *The Human Condition*. 2nd ed. Chicago: University of Chicago Press.

Aristotle. 1984. Politics. In *The Complete Works of Aristotle, Vol. 2*, ed. Jonathan Barnes. Trans. B. Jowett. Princeton: Princeton University Press.

Bradley, A.C. 1905. *Shakespearean Tragedy*. 2nd ed. London: Macmillan.

Butler, Judith. 1997. *The Psychic Life of Power*. Stanford: Stanford University Press.

Copjec, Joan. 2002. *Imagine There's No Woman: Ethics and Sublimation*, 128. Cambridge: MIT Press.

Kant, Immanuel. 2000. *Critique of the Power of Judgment*. Trans. Paul Guyer, and Eric Matthews. Cambridge: Cambridge University Press.

Lacan, Jacques. 2006. *Le Séminaire, Livre XVI: D'un Autre à l'Autre, 1968–1969*, ed. Jacques-Alain Miller. Paris: Seuil.

Patterson, Charles. 2002. *Eternal Treblinka: Our Treatment of Animals and the Holocaust*. New York: Lantern Books.

Sartre, Jean-Paul. 1956. *Being and Nothingness*. Trans. Hazel E. Barnes. New York: Washington Square Press.

Shakespeare, William. 1996. Othello. In *The Riverside Shakespeare*, 2nd ed. New York: Houghton Mifflin.

Beckett's 'Marionette Theater': Psychoanalysis, Ontological Violence, and the Language of Desubjectification in *Stories* and *The Unnamable*

Amanda Duncan

The Notion of Life in Beckett's Prose

In *Damned to Fame: The Life of Samuel Beckett*, James Knowlson explains how Beckett was known to ask his stage actors to read Kleist's essay 'On the Marionette Theater' as an illustration of the dramatic style he sought to capture in the 1970s' productions of *Happy Days* and the television play *Ghost Trio*. When recounting the essay to Roland Pickup, the principle actor in *Ghost Trio,* Beckett emphasized the beauty and grace of Kleist's puppets, whose movements, unburdened by human self-consciousness, are dictated by a series of pure mathematical permutations—a 'rhythm of movement,' 'around the center of gravity.'[1] When asked how such theater could be made possible, Beckett replied that 'the author had the duty to search for the perfect actor, that is, one who would have the ability to annihilate himself totally.' In Beckett's words, '[t]he best possible play is one in which there are no actors, only the text. I'm trying to write one.'[2]

A. Duncan (✉)
Pacific University, Forest Grove, OR, USA

G. Basu Thakur, J.M. Dickstein (eds.), *Lacan and the Nonhuman*,
The Palgrave Lacan Series, DOI 10.1007/978-3-319-63817-1_10

Beckett's determination to write what he considered to be the 'perfect' play—one in which language and action is unalloyed because it is radically free of its attachments to human self-consciousness—helps to explain the progression in his novels and short stories toward an almost mathematical purity of language; thus, the emphasis on character or plot gradually gives way to a nonrepresentational logic of postural movements, circuits, or positions. In a way analogous to Kleist's puppets, the human being in Beckett's experimental prose is incorporated into the text by way of gesture: Its bodily and verbal postures are placed in contact with forces that are internal to the impersonal vitalism or the 'life' of language itself.

By displacing self-present modes of expression onto the order of the Signifier's living autonomy, Beckett's postmodernism poses the questions: What is linguistic or textual 'life'? What is the 'human'? All the while he resists the urge to collapse these categories, as one of the 'voices' in Beckett's *Texts for Nothing* suggests: 'No need for a story, just a life, that's the mistake I made…to have wanted a story myself, whereas a life alone is enough.'[3] Beckett's rejection of the humanist model of subjectivity and life therefore confronts one with a paradox in which a 'life' is projected onto and played out technologically through language at the very point that marks the subject's disappearance into what the French psychoanalyst Jacques Lacan calls 'the Real'—a radically desubjectified 'beyond' of both language and human consciousness.

It is not unusual for modern philosophers and critics to draw connections between the aesthetic innovations of Samuel Beckett and those developed by twentieth-century nonrepresentational painters such as Jack Yeats and Francis Bacon. This connection is supported, in part, by Beckett's refusal to approach the Signifier as a means to communicate inner experience. As Beckett once said in conversation with Laurence Harvey: [W]ords are a form of complacency. …All you [have] to do [is] rearrange them and they express what you want'; 'if you really want to get down to the disaster, the slightest eloquence becomes unbearable. …[W]hat ever is said is so far from experience.'[4]

Beckett's wish to move away from what he describes to Harvey as a kind of aesthetic 'complacency' (i.e., referring to the way in which a representing subject substitutes a ready-made concept for what is becoming or in flux) helps to explain his interest in words or images that visibly fail to represent reality; and, in Beckett's words, that point 'directly' to themselves as a 'rupture in the lines of communication,' as a 'space that intervenes' in the Symbolic web of relations that construct meaning as a natural necessity.[5] This notion of 'direct' or nonrepresentational presentation constitutes for Beckett a form of resistance to the means-to-ends establishment of meaning, which he saw as a defining characteristic of hegemonic discourse. Indeed, Beckett consistently understands the function of modern art in terms of its obligation to introduce negativity, temporality, and movement into the notion of relation itself.

Beckett's interest in what we described earlier as a notion of 'direct' presentation becomes evident as early as his 1927 essay on James Joyce's *Work in Progress* (later to become *Finnegans Wake*), titled 'Dante...Bruno. Vico...Joyce.' In the essay, Beckett insists that any true art—as opposed to aesthetic forms enlisted in the service of ideological programs, popular in Nationalist Ireland and Germany at that time—begins in a sometimes painful or alienating splitting of the Signifier from its perceived attachment to the Symbol and its base in natural reality.

Emphasizing the importance of this absence of naturalized relations fundamental to aesthetic language, Beckett's essay attempts to revolutionize the way we see linguistic signs, such that the experience of a reader is no longer defined, as he says, by the intellectual operation of 'reading' the sign as a signifying unit. Accordingly, Beckett points to *Work in Progress* as a demonstration of the way that language can demand from the reader, as from the writer, a different way of experiencing the sign's 'sense.' Such an experience remains closely tied, according to Beckett, to the operations of metaphor and metonymy:

> Before articulation comes song; before abstract terms, metaphors. ...[In Joyce's work] form *is* content, content is form. ...It is not to be read—or rather it is not only to be read. It is to be looked at and listened to.[6]

In 'Dante...Bruno. Vico...Joyce,' Beckett rejects what he calls the 'metaphysical' approach to language, according to which the metaphor designates a self-present substitution of one relational term for another, and thus gains conceptual ground in an abstract or indirect, a priori relationship to Being. Whereas metaphysical language establishes these 'static' relations between words and things (i.e., subject and object) to secure referential truth and the illusion of authorial mastery, Joyce's modernism, according to Beckett, works by exposing the radical impossibility of an a priori relation itself. In other words, it bears witness to a gap, a difference or spacing that remains fundamental to the possibility of language.

Beckett thus traces the origin of 'poetic' language to a movement in which words break free of their means-to-ends arrangement in order to call attention to their 'primitive economic directness'—that is, as sensible 'things' that cannot be 'read' in the accepted sense, but rather 'looked at and listened to,' seen and sensed 'directly.'[7] To use Beckett's words, the 'primitive' metaphor involves 'force;' it is sense or meaning that 'insists' in language, or is produced physically, as a result of a particular kind of 'interior intertwining' or 'combination' of signs.[8] Moving beyond the metaphysical oppositions of interior and exterior, form and content, the poetic sign emerges as a figure for what Beckett calls, 'the exteriorization of thought' on the word 'surface.'[9] Implied in Beckett's model of signification therefore is a distinct notion of immanence: Human thought knots itself to the 'surface' movement of the Signifier as an exterior force, to which it must surrender its authority and self-presence.

Beckett's early critical essays bear witness to his concept of literature as the generation of textual meaning through a mechanical, even inhuman, metonymic 'slippage' of words and images—a movement of desire that transgresses the Symbolic laws of correspondence keeping representation stable, such as the principle of authorship that views the novel as a product of a self-conscious subjectivity. It is because of this approach to language that we might consider the proximity of Beckett's work to the psychoanalytic theory of Jacques Lacan who, like Beckett, also rejected the metaphysical notion of relation that establishes natural ties between the subject and object, the Signifier and the signified.[10]

As a student of the works of the linguists Ferdinand de Saussure and Roman Jakobson, Lacan insists that the Signifier can never 'hit' the signified. Forever barred from what he calls 'the Real,' the Signifier attains signification by reference to another Signifier via the operations of metonymy (i.e., displacement, association) and metaphor (i.e., condensation, substitution). What he opposes to the metaphysical concept of 'Being' and of our relation to it, is the notion that 'we are duped by *jouis-*

sance,' which is nothing but the 'Being of the signifier' and its meaning effects.[11] Every dimension of 'Being' therefore is produced by the limits of discourse; substance or origin is withdrawn (barred), and language can only work to manifest this inadequacy—this 'cut,' 'bar,' or 'gap' separating word and thing—over which Signifiers slip, qua link, into another reference.

Throughout his career, Lacan consistently points out how, for Freud, literature and dreams function as privileged domains in which the material Signifier—what Lacan calls 'the Letter'—signals this essential emptiness within itself. Like Beckett, Lacan turns repeatedly to Joyce's *Finnegans Wake* to draw attention to this impossibility of relation inherent in signification:

> What happens in Joyce's work? The signifier stuffs the signified. It is because the signifiers fit together, combine and concertina…that something is produced by way of meaning that may seem enigmatic, but is clearly closest to what we analysts have to read—slips of the tongue.[12]

In Seminar XX, Lacan describes how Joyce's signifiers 'stuff the signified,' an image that suggests how textual meaning, produced (as Lacan says) by a series of metonymic 'combinations' or surface interactions, 'above the bar,' is then 'injected,' as if retroactively, into the signified. In other words, Joyce's linguistic sleight-of-hand betrays the signified's inadequacy to ground meaning referentially in a natural origin. Lacan's linguistic metaphor therefore invokes an image from Joyce's *Ulysses* in which Leopold Bloom links language to music in as much as 'empty vessels make most noise.' For Lacan as for Joyce, words reach their maximal associative resonance—their 'fullness' of meaning—only when they evacuate referentially by subordinating human autonomy to the materiality of the Signifier and its inhuman movement or force.

Indeed, for Lacan this dehumanizing effect of language is precisely 'what is at stake' in the analytic setting, where words and chains of signifiers refuse to be 'read' or heard in the traditional sense, but slip into each other, 'combine and concertina'; they suggest themselves and, in doing so, point to an 'Other' dimension—a radical heteronomy gaping within human subjectivity.[13] For Lacan, the subject of the unconscious does not so much speak in language as it *is spoken*; language 'splits the subject' and opens within it a silent and inhuman passivity.

Accordingly, Joyce's postmodernism remains critically important to psychoanalysis because it bears witness to what Lacan calls, in 'The Instance of the Letter in the Unconscious,' a 'revolution' of language (in the sense in which we speak of the 'Copernican Revolution'), because what is called to question here is exactly the place man assigns himself as the center of his own conscious universe.[14] For although humanist thought grounds Being in the singular self-presence of consciousness, a fact best captured in the Cartesian mantra (i.e., '*cogito ergo sum*'), the subject of analytic discourse is displaced and split by its own language. It finds its truth in the Lacanian formula: 'I am thinking where I am not, therefore I am where I am not thinking. …I am not, where I am the plaything of my thought; I think about what I am where I do not think I am thinking.' Resonating with Beckett's fondness for puppets as a metaphor for the alienation central to being-in-language, the Symbolic order emerges in Lacan's work as a puppet master to which, 'I am more attached than to myself, since, at the most assented to heart of my identity to myself, he pulls the strings.'[15]

The 1927 publication of 'Dante…Bruno. Vico…Joyce' was followed almost 20 years later by a torrential period of creative production in Beckett's life; it manifested itself in the brilliant, but much neglected, *Stories*. Published in 1946, the 'The End' and 'The Expelled,' both contained in the collection, are commonly read as preparatory pieces in anticipation of Beckett's well-known *The Trilogy* (*Molloy, Malone Dies*). What ties these works together is the unmistakable presence of an endless and often debilitating interrogation of the subject's power over his or her own speech; each bear heavily on a series of problems that lie at the center of the text's production: The contradiction, for instance, between the intentional aims of the author and the uncontrollable difference that the expressive 'vehicle' produces on its own within the exigencies of human expression.

As gestural articulations of this contradiction, the principle characters of 'The End' and 'The Expelled' are wandering figures, ones who are perpetually in transport, and who have been deprived of a home, a name, or origin, and even the anthropomorphizing features of the face. The lack of humanizing features expected of literary characters is intensified by the fact that Beckett favors the nonrelational, textual, or mechanical processes that underpin writing—what Lacan calls 'the Letter'—over the mimetic effects of story or background. Having forgone both characterization and plot, what is staged in the *Stories* is precisely what Beckett previously described as the nonanthropomorphic 'life' of language (i.e., a rhythm of movement) played out in and through the 'surface' of signs. In this way, Beckett's homeless figures are themselves images of the Signifier's transgression beyond the home-centered economy of human meaning that ties them to signifieds.

Both stories thus begin with a scene of 'expulsion' from the home, and Beckett continues to play on all the possibilities or permutations of this word in its related senses of 'abandonment' and loss such as 'excess,' 'excrement,' 'birth' and 'creation':

> I set off...extraordinary splaying of the feet to the right and to the left. ...A policeman stopped me. ...He said 'if you can't bloody well get about like everyone else, you might as well stay at home.'...And that he should attribute to me a home was no small satisfaction.[16]

Whereas, in 'Dante...Bruno. Vico...Joyce,' Beckett testifies to the fact that it is by means of the vehicle's anthropomorphic identity with the Symbolic Law of referentiality that language establishes its dominating presence, the *Stories* begin to trace the movement of a figure, one who is *lawless* in this respect, whose 'wild' and 'defective' force prevents it from ever being 'assimilated to [a] category' or 'home' ('it always ended in the same way, I mean, in a loss of equilibrium followed by a fall. ...The widest sidewalk is never enough for me, once I set myself in motion'[17]).

Indeed, once it has 'set itself in motion,' the figure keeps slipping away from a solid ground on which to regain linguistic 'equilibrium,' away from the relational exigencies of narrative structure that work to 'police' or control meaning, by bringing it to a determinate 'end.' Thus, the wandering figure finds himself in the situation of being, as Beckett says, unable to put his wandering 'to a stop,' unable to transcend an essential passivity in order make himself 'useful'—'to put himself to work' within the textual unfolding of meaning.

This ontological problem unleashes a series of preoccupations that persist throughout Beckett's novels: What, for example, does it mean for the imagination to 'inhabit' its linguistic vehicle? How does the subject limit the movement of its own signification or bring it to an end? Where is the beginning or origin of the work located? At one point, the wandering figure of 'The End' does find temporary rest in a wooden shed. Withdrawn into its shelter on a bed of ferns, he awakens from sleep to find himself in the 'uncanny' position of being, as he says, 'immobile' and yet still in 'transport'—immobile and yet still unable to escape from the inhuman momentum of the Signifier, that has generated him:

> One day I could not get up. The cow saved me. Goaded by the icy mist she came in search of me…she dragged me across the threshold and out into the giant streaming ferns, where I was forced to let go. …More master of myself I might have made a friend of her.[18]

What is remarkable about the image in this passage is its proximity to the zero level of its own ontological production. What we are presented with is an image of the work's being made, of creation, 'expulsion' or birth—an image of language as it struggles to separate itself from an authorial or conceptual plan. In addition, it is for this reason that the figure in Beckett's story cannot so much transport himself (or his idea) via the vehicle but is transported passively by language as an inhuman power, envisioned in the image of the silent and speechless life of the animal.

'More master' of himself, as Beckett writes, the figure might have found a way to stop this movement to forcibly bring his idea 'to work' within literary language. But the truth of Beckett's literature is that of its material production, which demands that literary language remain (unlike the anthropomorphic language of utility), a place of abandonment and refusal: 'But in the end she prevailed. For she dragged me across the threshold and out into the giant streaming ferns, where I was forced to let go.'

Literary language is not, for Beckett, a 'vehicle' of human subjectification: Unable to stop the movement of figuration to bring thought to work in language as a transcendental entity, the imagination encounters its vehicle as a nonrelational image, which Beckett calls a 'threshold,' in the face of which the figure is 'forced to let go' of its own signifying rules or principles. Two lines cross and are linked together, the artist and the work; neither are without the other, both 'cling' together in a double movement that is nonidentical or is at variance with itself. This is also to say that the Signifier can only be said to support the imagination by 'dragging' it, as Beckett writes, beyond its own human limits.

Beckett's *Stories* thus begins to delimit a point in his career in which, as he wrote in 'Dante...Bruno. Vico...Joyce': '[T]he exteriorization of thought' is transformed into the work's point of departure. 'The End' is one such work that, accordingly, begins with its own dissolution: Its possibility remains located at the point where, as the narrator says, 'the words desert you' and 'the vessels stop communicating.' Yet this movement in which the vehicle 'abandons,' 'deserts,' and destroys its passenger is also the passage through which the work becomes realized.

This aporia becomes self-reflexive in the story's last lines: 'The memory came faint and cold of a story I might have told in the likeness of my life, I mean without the courage to end or the strength to go on.'[19] In this ellipsis, through which the work opens itself to the bottomless law of its own double movement, the sign forgoes its functional relationship to action, utility, or self-consciousness, favoring instead the limit toward which it is drawn—the threshold in which the actualization of meaning is suspended in a sea of indeterminacy.

Language and Violence

In 'Language, Violence and Nonviolence,' Slavoj Žižek questions the conventional, humanist view of language as a medium of harmonious, nonviolent reconciliation: 'What if,' he asks, 'humans exceed animals in their capacity for violence precisely because they speak?'[20] Žižek recollects that it was Martin Heidegger who first elaborated this problem on the ontological level when he rejected the traditional idea of 'essence' (Wesen) as a stable core of Being, favoring instead the notion of essence as a verb ('essencing') or process ('*Wesen der Sprache*')—a disclosure of Being that occurs in and through language, the 'house of being.'[21]

In *Introduction to Metaphysics*, for example, Heidegger links the founding gesture of poetry to a violent disclosure of Being in which our old world comes out of joint, so to speak, and loses its balance as a new Symbolic universe is formed. Žižek, nevertheless, points out a violent aspect of language that is absent in the preceding formulation—a Lacanian 'twist' to Heidegger's notion of language as the 'house of being,' which supports and sustains the human animal. That is, what Heidegger overlooks is precisely what Lacan calls the 'Real of jouissance'—the 'traumatic impact of the very "passivity" of being caught in language,' the irremediable abyss between the subject and language, the play between the human and animal.

In Žižek's words, 'the human animal doesn't "fit" language [but is] tortured, mutilated'; it emerges there as 'the Thing or that part/aspect of the real which suffers from the signifier.'[22] Never at home in its own home, caught up and played out in the 'torture-house' of language and its signifying effects, the Lacanian subject survives as an irreparable gap in the Symbolic field, a 'cut in the order of Being in which the real of jouissance breaks in.'[23] In this way, Lacan grasps what Heidegger's formulation overlooks as 'the most radical zero-point of the Cartesian cogito,' 'the point of the negative intersection between being and thinking,' 'the vanishing point at which…I am reduced to a void in the order of being.'[24]

It is perhaps useful to understand many of Samuel Beckett's stories and plays as taking, as their point of departure, something very close to this 'zero-point of the Cartesian cogito'—that is, the negative intersection between being and thinking, human and animal. Indeed, it is helpful, even, to work through some key aspects of Beckett's prose with a mind to the relationship between language and ontological violence. The most sustained, even indefatigable exploration of this relationship between language and violence can be found in Beckett's 1953 *The Unnamable,* which clearly takes as its theme the refusal of the Signifier to 'house' authorial presence, the torment and shame of signification, the mutilation or splitting required of the subject as it enters the Symbolic order. The novel, which abandons even the pretense of narrative or story, stages the production of meaning as a form of ontological violence that forces the one who speaks into a relationship with that part of itself that remains strangely absent or inhuman: It reduces the speaker to the status of a 'Thing' or a nonhuman 'creature'—a 'worm.'

Rather than authenticate self-presence, in *The Unnamable* it is precisely this capacity for speech that dehumanizes the subject, who can only come into being by disappearing from his statement. More specifically, the novel works untiringly to foreground the impossibility of speaking without the metonymic movement of displacement having already 'ventriloquized' the subject, as Beckett's 'creature' suggests: 'It is they who have stuffed me full of these groans that choke me. And out of which all pours unchanged, I have only to belch to be sure of hearing them, the same old sour teachings I can't change a title of. A parrot, that's what they're up against, a parrot.'[25]

The aporia central to *The Unnamable* therefore originates in the fact that the nameless 'Thing' who inhabits the torture house of the text is 'obliged to live' and 'condemned to speak' in words and voices that can never be assumed. Since, for Beckett as for Lacan, Being or substance is constituted nonrelationally, in and by the Signifier, this impossibility of appropriating the movement of discourse is articulated in terms of the creature's failure to assume its own principle of life, its inevitable inability to know whether or not the meaning effects of language—all these 'signs of life'—go along 'outside of me' or 'without me' or whether they are the very thing I am ('It all boils down to a question of words. ...I have to speak a certain way...first of the creature that I am not, as if I were he, and then, as if I were he, of the creature that I am').[26]

Exiled in its own language, the subject of Beckett's work occupies a place that analytic discourse calls 'ex-timacy': It can only 'testify' to its being a subject in terms of what it calls the 'language of the other':

> [W]ords falling, you don't know where, you don't know whence. ...I'll have said it inside me, then in the same breath outside me, perhaps what I feel, an outside and an inside and me in the middle, perhaps that what I am, the thing that divides me in the middle.[27]

Mutilated or split by its own language, never managing to actualize itself in its own discourse, the subject of *The Unnamable* appears in writing as a 'partition' or fold. It is itself pure difference; it is 'the thing that divides':

'I'm the partition, I've two surfaces, and no thickness, perhaps that's what I feel, myself vibrating, I'm the tympanum, on the one hand the mind, on the other the world, I don't belong to either.'[28]

In this way, Beckett's *The Unnamable* offers an image of subjectivity and authorship as an essential displacement or spacing—a simultaneous withdrawal/presenting of Being; the double movement or intersection between concealment and disclosure, light and darkness, in which meaning violently irrupts. Nevertheless, perhaps we could do no better than to conceive of subjectivity in language terms of what Beckett describes as a 'vibration' or the 'convulsive space' of the threshold itself, pictured beautifully in the following lines from his 'Quatre Poèmes': '[M]y peace is there in the receding mist/when I may cease from treading these long shifting thresholds/and live the space of a door/that opens and shuts.'[29]

Notes

1. James Knowlson, *Dammed to Fame: The Life of Samuel Beckett* (New York: Grove Press, 1996), p. 558; Heinrich von Kleist, 'On the Marionette Theater,' trans. Idris Parry. In Amos Leslie Willson, ed., *German Romantic Criticism, Vol. 21* (London/New York: Continuum, 1982), p. 239
2. Deirdre Bair, *Samuel Beckett: A Biography*, 1st Summit Books ed. (New York: Summit; distributed by Simon & Schuster, 1990), p. 554.
3. Samuel Beckett and S. E. Gontarski, *Samuel Beckett: The Complete Short Prose, 1929–1989*, 1st ed. (New York: Grove Press, 1995), p. 119.
4. Erik Tonning, *Samuel Beckett's Abstract Drama: Works for Stage and Screen, 1962–1985, Vol. 10* (Bern, Switzerland: Peter Lang, 2007), p. 266
5. Samuel Beckett and Ruby Cohn, *Disjecta: Miscellaneous Writings and a Dramatic Fragment.* (London: J. Calder, 1983), p. 70.
6. Ibid. pp. 24, 27–28.
7. Ibid., p. 29.
8. Ibid., pp. 22, 29.
9. Ibid., p. 29.
10. It is worth noting that Beckett underwent a course of psychoanalysis with Wilfred Bion at the Tavstock Clinic in London between the years

of 1934–1935. During this time Beckett read extensively on psychoanalysis and took detailed, typewritten notes on works by Otto Rank, Wilhelm Stekel, Ernst Jones, and Sigmund Freud, among others. See Knowlson, *Dammed to Fame,* p. 172.

11. Jacques Lacan. *On Feminine Sexuality: The Limits of Love and Knowledge* (New York: W. W. Norton, 1998), p. 70.
12. Lacan, ibid., pp. 34, 36–37. Bruce Fink's footnote for this passage reads: 'Here, signifier is injected into the signified, apparently like fuel is injected into an engine,' p. 34.
13. Much like Joyce, Lacan plays on the musical characteristics of language. As a verb, the word 'concertina' means 'to cause to fold or collapse in the manner of a concertina,' 'a musical instrument resembling an accordion, played by stretching and squeezing between the hands' (Oxford English Dictionary).
14. Jacques Lacan and Bruce Fink. *Ecrits: A Selection* (New York: W. W. Norton, 2002), p. 156.
15. Ibid., p. 163.
16. Samuel Beckett, *Samuel Beckett: The Grove Centenary Edition, Vol. IV: Poems, Short Fiction, Criticism* (New York: Grove Press, 2006), p. 252.
17. Ibid.
18. Ibid., p. 285.
19. Ibid., p. 290.
20. Slavoj Žižek, 'Language, Violence and Nonviolence.' *International Journal of Žižek Studies* 2(1–12): 2, 2016.
21. Ibid., p. 3.
22. Ibid., p. 5.
23. Ibid., p. 9.
24. Ibid., p. 10.
25. Samuel Beckett and Patrick Bowles, *Three Novels: Molloy; Malone Dies; The Unnamable* (New York: Grove Press, 2009), p. 335.
26. Ibid.
27. Ibid., pp. 382–383.
28. Ibid.
29. Beckett (2006), p. 39.

Bibliography

Bair, Deirdre. 1990. *Samuel Beckett: A Biography*, 1st Summit Books ed. New York: Summit; distributed by Simon & Schuster.

Beckett, Samuel. 2006. *Samuel Beckett: The Grove Centenary Edition, Vol. IV: Poems, Short Fiction, Criticism*. New York: Grove Press.

Beckett, Samuel, and Patrick Bowles. 2009. *Three Novels: Molloy; Malone Dies; The Unnamable*. New York: Grove Press.

Beckett, Samuel, and Ruby Cohn. 1983. *Disjecta: Miscellaneous Writings and a Dramatic Fragment*. London: J. Calder.

Beckett, Samuel, and S.E. Gontarski. 1995. *Samuel Beckett: The Complete Short Prose, 1929–1989*. 1st ed. New York: Grove Press.

Heidegger, Martin. 1953 (rev. 2014). *Introduction to Metaphysics*. Trans. Richard Polt and Gregory Fried. New Haven: Yale Univeristy Press.

Knowlson, James. 1996. *Dammed to Fame: The Life of Samuel Beckett*. New York: Grove Press.

Lacan, Jacques. 1998. *On Feminine Sexuality: The Limits of Love and Knowledge*. New York: W. W. Norton.

Lacan, Jacques, and Bruce Fink. 2002. *Ecrits: A Selection*. New York: W. W. Norton.

Tonning, Erik. 2007. *Samuel Beckett's Abstract Drama: Works for Stage and Screen, 1962–1985 Vol. 10*. Oxford: Peter Lang.

Žižek, Slavoj. 2016. Language, Violence and Nonviolence. *International Journal of Žižek Studies* 2(3).

Do Electric Sheep Dream of Androids?: On the Place of Fantasy in Consideration of the Nonhuman

Calum Neill

The standard objection to Object Oriented Ontology is as simple as it is, apparently, devastating. How can one conceive of the object without the subject? Grammatically speaking, clearly one cannot. The 'one' here *is* the subject which necessarily, conceptually, precedes the object it would conceive. The counter to this dismissal might be something along the lines of Nietzsche's famous refutation of the *cogito*.[1] For Nietzsche, the apparently subjective 'it' which is taken to be doing the conceiving here is not obviously reducible to the conventional conception we would have of a subject, an *I*. Moreover, Nietzsche draws our attention to the fact that grammatical structure already assumes a particular process at work. The way of speaking smuggles in a thinking of the world and how that world might function. We assume thinking to be an activity and that driving any activity there must be an actor. When an object is conceived, there must be a conceiver doing the conceiving. If we retrace the Cartesian logic in response to which this point is made, and thus from which this thinking emerges, we return to an asubjective happening. It thinks. It

C. Neill (✉)
Edinburgh Napier University, Edinburgh, UK

G. Basu Thakur, J.M. Dickstein (eds.), *Lacan and the Nonhuman*,
The Palgrave Lacan Series, DOI 10.1007/978-3-319-63817-1_11

conceives. Or simply there is conception. For there to be a conception of an object, that object must be conceived. Let's leave aside the problematic 'one' sneaked in as actor and leave the work of conception untethered. A simple tautology. The paradox here is that the Nietzschean intervention, while providing a productive lesson on the error of servitude to grammar, leaves the object just as enchained a phenomenon. Even if we problematize the ontology of the subject, the noumenal object remains just as out of reach. We bracket or renounce the doer but the object is no less rooted in the doing. Even if there is no knower knowing the known, the known, to be known, must still be known.

Early in his career Lacan was keen to warn us to be wary of any philosophy "directly issuing from the Cogito".[2] It is clear from both 'The Mirror Stage as Formative of the Function of the *I* in Psychoanalytic Experience' and from the many subsequent and productive references Lacan makes to Descartes[3] that this warning is no simple call to reject Descartes' project. The emphasis in Lacan's statement is very much on the 'directly'. What Lacan wants to advance is a thinking of the subject which takes Descartes seriously but avoids the isolationism which hampers the project from the beginning. Just as Descartes' world always remains a world beyond, so the heirs of Descartes remain trapped in a subject-object relation which always tends to subsume the latter under the former. The Nietzschean solution discussed above, its radicality notwithstanding, still retains a reasonably straightforward subject-object paradigm, albeit one in which the subject is divested of any agency. What Lacan allows us to think is a manner of conceiving the subject-object relation which neither abandons the subject as an archaic inconvenience nor relegates the object to an always already ancillary status. Whether the subject *is* a thinking thing, as Descartes asserted,[4] or it is an effect, a phenomenal model, as an apparent anti-Cartesian like Metzinger would hold,[5] the experience of what we might, however erroneously, call consciousness persists.

What Lacan allows us to think is a paradigm wherein subjects and objects persist but where one is not collapsed into a manifestation or effect of the other, where neither precedes the other. We can appreciate the beginnings of this logic in 'The Mirror Stage' where the becoming subject finds itself before another and, through this encounter, finds itself in the already unfolding experience of an always failing process of identification. The process is always failing for the simple reason that that with which the becoming subject has begun to identify is not itself and, thus, the self that the becoming subject is in the process of forging is necessarily alien. The self it takes itself to be is predicated on an identity with something other than itself. Its self is other. The becoming subject finds what it mistakes to be itself on the basis of a misidentification with a hazy object, an object to which it then works to add clarity through a continuance of this process, resulting in what we might term a productive infinite regress. Neither the subject nor the object can stand alone. Each is forged through the encounter with the other. Which means too, then, that neither has claim to a primacy.

What we can understand from this logic of becoming is that the subject—in terms of its own grasping or positing of itself, its self-model, the formation of the *I* function—always consists in something outside of (what it would take to be) itself. A similar fate befalls the object. We are not, however, talking here of a symmetry. It is not, as for Hegel in his famous dialectic of the Lord and the Bondsman, a situation where each partner in the dyad has before it another self-consciousness, mirroring it in all substantive regards.[6] Hegel's description, fruitful as it may be, necessarily assumes a God-like view. For Lacan there is no symmetry, no possibility of an exterior vantage point. What this means, then, is that while the subject comes to model itself on a mistaken identification with the object it has before it, comes to introject aspects of the object, the object comes to be adorned and hewed through this same selective identification. The subject sees itself in the object and it sees the object in itself. There is no point zero for this operation.

The theory Lacan is weaving here not only allows a conception of subjectivity without ground, which is arguably Lacan's primary point at this stage, but it allows us to grasp the fact that the subject cannot stand apart from the object. This is perhaps most clearly seen in Lacan's 1960 essay 'The Subversion of the Subject and the Dialectic of Desire in the Freudian Unconscious' where, in developing his graphic depiction of the structure of the subject, in all its rich and temporally challenging complexity, he posits the subject as an idea framed in response to a questioning of and from an Other and, in so positing the subject, he straps it to an object.[7]

Cloven by language, alien to itself, constitutionally incomplete—both in the structural and the temporal senses that that would imply—the subject *is* not, except insofar as it posits itself as *to be*, and that which will allow it to (impossibly) be is necessarily another. This other, the objective correlate of the subject, is what allows the movement of desire which sustains the subject.

This, of course, is the formula of fantasy; the subject in relation to *a*. The *a* here had originally been meant to indicate the partial object, in a development of Kleinian theory,[8] but by 1960 it had taken on a more nuanced and slippier sense, operating algebraically to refuse any easy coaption to any preconceived notions. Lacan was well aware that the other (the *autre*, of which the *a* might be understood as the erstwhile synecdoche) is never itself a subject, that the other is always another for a subject, while the subject is always a retroactively produced effect of language. This would be to say that, while the subject is an aphanitic pulsion, emerging from and being lost to language, the other is always an object. The logic of objecthood here is one already noted by Descartes when he peers down from his window at the people in the street below and questions how he knows they are people and not automatons dressed as people.[9] For Lacan, and arguably already for Descartes, the point is obvious; we do not. Each other we encounter is as other to us as any automaton. The other is met as an object. What is interesting is the various ways in which we invest and pump this object with attributes and affects which convince us otherwise. That is to say, what is interesting is the way in which the mode of fantasy connects us libidinally to an object.

Around the time Lacan was utilising his graph of desire as a mechanism to unfold a dynamic theory of subjectivity, he was also immersed in a developing discourse on ethics. In this context, in his seventh seminar, he seeks, as it might seem he would have to, to account for precisely this dissymmetry of the subject and the other. Focusing on a passage from Freud's *A Project for a Scientific Psychology*,[10] Lacan draws our attention to the way in which Freud disentangles the different modes through which we take in the other.[11] In Freud's original text, the other in question is the mother, and specifically the mother's breast (i.e. the other as partial object, *objet a*). The point Lacan extracts from this, however, is general.

Whenever we encounter another, we do so in three modes. There is that in the other which presents as known, either in the sense that it is graspable, comprehendible, or in the sense that it is familiar. To be familiar would to be suggest that something has been encountered before. In having been encountered before, or in so seeming to resemble something which has been encountered before, the familiar is that with which we identify. It is already a part of our psychic makeup and thus already part of the complex of what we take ourselves to be. This imaginary component is always accompanied by a symbolic component, a structure of knowledge into which the familiar fits or into which the unfamiliar can be fitted, rendering it now familiar. Of course, where there is the imaginary and the symbolic, there is also the real. In this context, this might be understood as the incomprehensible or simply not comprehended, that which does not fit.

It is easy to see then, how, in the context of the encounter with the human other, we grasp the other human on the basis of a degree of familiarity, both in the sense of identification and in the sense of coaption to prescripted knowledge. When Descartes gazes at the bodies moving in the street below and simultaneously questions and assumes their identity as people like himself, he is operating on this basis. Not only can he draw on his intellect but he is drawing on a felt identification with his fellow citizens and the assumption that they are more or less like himself. If we take Descartes' question more at his word, however, and assume Santpoort to have been populated by sophisticated robots, Lacan's structure of comprehension remains in place. There is that in the robot with which we can identify, there is that in the robot which we can understand and there is that in the robot which escapes both these mechanisms and yet imposes itself nonetheless.

This accounts for not only the uncanny affect of automatons, their coupling of the familiar and the unfamiliar,[12] but also for the persistent questioning of their status in fiction and film. Although Frank L Baum's *Tik-tok*[13] is not endowed with what we would normally understand as human agency, he is presented as having a para-human form and this form is enough to engender identification. A few years later, in Čapek's *R.U.R.*,[14] the robots are given an interiority which exceeds the mechanical and they then begin to develop what is presented as human affect. By the time of Ridley Scott's *Bladerunner*[15] or Alex Garland's *Ex Machina*[16] it is the robot's own questioning of their status which is pushed to the foreground. *Bladerunner* is quintessential here in that it plays out through the robots or replicants what is essentially the core question of Descartes' *Meditations*: the existence or not of the self. Roy Batty's famous 'Tears in the Rain' speech encapsulates the core tension which runs through the film. The assumed essence of self is presented as predicated on memory but when those memories are shown to be false and unveiled as implants, then does this consequently remove the essence of self? The question is one of knowledge and dumb fact. The dumb fact is that, within the world of *Bladerunner*, the replicants are not human, they are biorobots, artefacts. Nonetheless, it is possible for a replicant to experience existence and to supplement implanted memories with actual memories and it is possible for a replicant to believe that it is human. This is the core tension. Does belief alter the facticity of the experience of being human? Can the difference between the human and the nonhuman be brought down to a question of belief? Roy Batty knows full well that he is an artefact, programmed to die at a set point. Rachel on the contrary is a replicant but does not know it, and when she is told, she struggles to believe or accept this knowledge. Deckard is the final piece of the puzzle. Where we, the apparently all seeing spectator, know that Roy and Rachel are replicants, we are left unsure of Deckard's status, with various hints pushing us to the conclusion that he is a replicant but without this being unambiguously established.[17] Roy knows and believes that he is a replicant. Rachel knows but does not fully accept/believe that she is a replicant. Deckard neither knows nor believes that he is a replicant. All three, however, are invested with a desire, for life, for connection, for something akin to a human existence.

The point is not, then, the difference between the three characters, the truth of their status. The point is rather the truth the film reflects back to us. Just as Lacan posits the formula of fantasy as a response to the question, *Che vuoi?* so, then, it is the fantasy we construct in response to the film which tells us something about ourselves, and about our desire. The other here is posited as almost human, nonhuman but human enough to open a gap to mirror the gap we experience in our own self-experience. When Roy Batty reminisces about the "C-beams glitter[ing] in the dark near the Tannhäuser Gate",[18] he provides us with a vivid example of what Meillassouix terms "the great outdoors".[19] In explicating the "paradox of the arche-fossil"[20] Meillassouix is concerned with what can be known about that which has never offered itself up as the object of experience. The implication in Batty's speech is that he, as a replicant, has travelled to parts of the universe unexplored by human beings, and, thus, has experienced things that human beings have not experienced. His speech then raises the question of the value of such experiences. They cannot be transmitted in such a way that would render them concrete for the human interlocutor and, therefore, must die with Roy. All we can do is imagine the C-beams, paint our own picture of their glittering. We cannot match Batty's memory to our own. But, then, is this really any different from our interactions with (what we take to be) other human beings?

Arguably what Batty describes is the fate of all experience and the failure of all communication. Not only is what is experienced put into words but it is always already filtered and forged in words. The very things which are abstracted as experience are grasped as such on the basis of language. When we seek to then grasp someone else's account of an experience, we necessarily do so on the basis of a shared linguistic repertoire and on a purely presumed and prior shared experience. Roy Batty's experience of the Tannhäuser Gate is no more beyond my ken than my grandfather's experience of watching whales in the northern Atlantic or indeed my wife's experience of watching *Bladerunner*. No more so, but no less so. Experience is necessarily shaped by the symbolic. Communication is necessarily stained by the imaginary.

The fundamental fantasy here is that there is a commonality to human experience, that both that which is experienced is experienced in common and that that which is not directly experienced in common can be transmitted, more or less efficiently, through language or art.

There is a core point, then, that emerges from Lacan's theory and allows us to appreciate an often overlooked issue with the entire notion of the post- or non-human, whether it is reaching out into the great outdoors and speculating on that which is beyond us or working to unsettle an archaic anthropocentrism.

When, in the context of discussing the possibility of the post-human subject, Rosi Braidotti dismisses the Lacanian symbolic as "out-dated",[21] comparing it to a "Polaroid shot of world which has since moved on", she is missing something vital in the Lacanian theory of the subject. Braidotti consigns Lacan to the past, arguing that his model of the subject was already becoming irrelevant in the 1970s. Her mistake is both in thinking that Lacan's notion of the symbolic is primary and that, in its primacy, it is predicated on a fixed notion of "family and other inter-subjective relations". Braidotti wants to argue that the world has changed and that such changes have produced radical new modes of what she terms "inter-subjective relationality". The terminology here is crucial. Braidotti retains a notion of inter-subjectivity which Lacan had abandoned back in the 1950s.[22] The problem with the term 'inter-subjective' is that is assumes precisely the God's eye view that Lacan had already found problematic in Hegel in the 1940s.[23] An inter-subjective model would be one in which there is an assumed symmetry, two comparable entities, each endowed with a subjective interiority. Not only was Lacan eager to disturb this notion of interiority but, despite the influence of Merleau-Ponty, Lacan's work from early on runs thoroughly counter to the phenomenological notion of grasping the other by analogy.[24] Where for Husserl the best we can do is grasp the other on the basis of an analogy with ourselves, for Lacan this is the pitfall of imaginary identification, which precisely stops me seeing the other as other and allows me to overwrite the other with myself. As discussed above, Lacan argues that each encounter with the other entails three modes: a symbolic mode, an imaginary mode and a real mode. It is not simply the insistence of the later which is crucial here but the insistence of the latter in its inseparability from the other two modes. This is what sets Lacan radically apart from the phenomenologists on this point.

For Braidotti, Lacan's theory misses the novelty of late capitalism and the possibilities and modes of inter-relation this moment in history creates. Rightly she draws attention to the problems of psychological essentialism which accompany the refusal of contemporary modes of being in the world, the idea that the human subject simply is, as an essentially atomistic entity, and that novel connections and ways of grasping the world and ourselves are mere appendages forming attributes which do not fundamentally shape or affect what we are. It is such an essentialist perspective which would endorse as common sense the subject-object divide which object oriented and speculative realist perspectives would seek to problematize. Braidotti's mistake is in thinking Lacan sits on the essentialist side of this argument. Far from it, Lacan's notion of the subject refuses essentialism from the outset, portraying a subject which is rather inessential, inadequate to itself, which is posited on a mistaken encounter with something beyond itself and is ever-fading from its own sights.

Lacan's notion of the symbolic, imaginary and real describe a structure of experience which is meant to allow us the possibility of grasping a notion of subjectivity which refuses to be grasped. The theory, like the subject it seeks to offer up, falters on its own impossibility. Reading Lacan (the late Lacan in particular) is an experience of reading a theory which unwrites itself as it is written, much in the same way as the Lacanian subject disappears under the signifier which would seek to articulate it.[25] It is evident in a seminar like *The Sinthome*[26] that Lacan is very aware of the impossibility of describing the very thing he is trying to describe without at the same time contradicting himself. The result is a giddy, vibrant theory of an impossibly impossible experience, a subjectivity which cannot be grasped and yet cannot not insist.

Far from a notion of subjectivity which is "forever static in a historical limbo,"[27] Lacan's is a notion of subjectivity which is structurally incomplete in the most radical sense and thus constitutionally open, even if it does not know this itself. In terms of self-grasping, the most the Lacanian subject can hope for is an always inadequate, retroactive positing of what might have been. Where for Braidotti this is a "mournful vision of a subject desperately attached to the conditions of its own impotence" and, as such, "is quite simply an inadequate representation of what we are in the process of becoming", Lacan's theory allows us a more nuanced perspective. From a Lacanian perspective this is not a vision of the subject at all. It is a necessarily failed theory of the subject, a theory of the subject which knows from the outset that just as, and in part because, the subject itself is failed, so too the theory which strives to be adequate to this subject must also fail. But importantly the notion of failure here is one which allows for an ever closer circulation of the void of impossibility, ever closer but always still infinitely far.

The vision of the subject that post-humanists like Braidotti advance is a vision of the subject thrust into the future, a vision of the subject as what it might be becoming or what it may be; a romantically vague notion of a nomadic warrior forever, although perhaps productively, out of synch with our contemporary experience. Lacan's name for such a vision is fantasy. This is not to belittle such a vision. Any positing of the subject is subject to a similar charge, if charge indeed it is. Lacan's point is that all we can do is posit ourselves in fantasy or, phrased otherwise, all fantasy should be understood as, no matter what it is a fantasy of, a fantasmatic positing of the subject. We cannot know the nonhuman without in some way relating it to ourselves simply because whatever we grasp we grasp on the basis of ourselves, although never completely. In a similar way we can never grasp ourselves except on the basis of our already forged encounters with that which exceeds us. Nonhuman counterparts like the replicants allow us an appreciation of the iterative and ultimately failing logic of any such grasping.

Our inclination to anthropomorphise the other, whether it is the animal other or the machinic other, coupled with our occasional awareness that this is what we do, lures us into an age-old trap. From polar bears savaging seals to ants building intricate constructions, from bacteria to hurricanes, from replicants to malfunctioning vacuum cleaners, our discourses imbue the nonhuman with human inclinations, motivations, intentions. The logic here, the logic we are vaguely aware of, is that we model, and thus master, the nonhuman world on the basis of an analogy with ourselves. We see the polar bear as human-like, although we know the comparison only stretches so far. We comprehend bacteria in terms of human warfare and invasion because gives us a basis on which to begin to think what is going on. We see ourselves in Deckard and his uncertainty over what he is, although we know our predicament is not actually his. Or do we? The final flaw in the temptation to anthropomorphise is not that we read human traits into the nonhuman so much as we read them into the human. We assume that there is a core to be being human in the first place that sets us apart when, just as we anthropomorphise the nonhuman other, so too do we anthropomorphise the human other and so too do we anthropomorphise ourselves.

The title of the original Philip K. Dick novella on which the film *Bladerunner* is based, *Do Androids Dream of Electric Sheep?*[28] appears to be raising a question of the essence or unicity of the human. If a replicant, an android, can form memories, then can they experience desire? If they dream, is their dream version of themselves like but not like our dream version of ourselves? If we, as desiring organisms, dream of organic sheep, do they as machines dream of machinic sheep? In contemplating this, we should keep in mind that the posited electric sheep is a dream dreamt by a dreamt dreamer, and this dreaming is the fantasy of a self, itself posited as fantasy. The Lacanian point which would then emerge here is the question of the locus of the subject, however aphanitic, who cannot but assume responsibility for the fantasy. There is no already forged answer here, no truth to this question. Rather it is the question of the subject itself. Who dreams the dream of the electric sheep? Who posits the subject you might be? Who dreams they are not a replicant? Do you?

Notes

1. Nietzsche, F. (2001) Beyond Good and Evil, trans. J. Norman. Cambridge: Cambridge University Press. pp. 17–18.
2. Lacan, J. (2006) 'The Mirror Stage as Formative of the *I* Function as Revealed in Psychoanalytic Experience' in Lacan, J. (2006) *Écrits: The First* Complete Edition in English, trans. B. Fink. London: Norton. pp. 75–81.
3. E.g. Lacan, J. (1977/1973) The Four Fundamental Concepts of Psychoanalysis, trans. A. Sheridan. London: Penguin.
4. Descartes, R. (2014) *Meditations on First Philosophy*. Cambridge. CUP. p. 19.
5. Mettzinger, T. (2003) *Being No One: The Self-Model Theory of Subjectivity.* Cambridge, MA. MIT Press.
6. Hegel, G.W.F. (1967) *The Phenomenology of Mind*, trans. J.B. Baillie. New York: Harper and Row. p. 229.
7. Lacan, J. (1977), 'Subversion of the Subject and Dialectic of Desire' in Lacan, J. (1977) Écrits: The First Complete Edition in English, trans. B. Fink. London: Norton. p. 690.
8. Lacan, J. (1998) *Séminaire, tome 4: la Relation d'objet*. Paris. Seuil.

9. Descartes, R. (2014) Meditations on First Philosophy. Cambridge. CUP. p. 21
10. Freud, S. (1966) A Project for a Scientific Psychology in The Complete Works of Sigmund Freud, Vol.1: Pre-Psychoanalytical Publications and Unpublished Drafts, trans. J. Strachey. London: Hogarth. p. 331.
11. Lacan, J (1992) The Ethics of Psychoanalysis: The Seminar of Jacques Lacan, Book VII, 1959–1960, trans. D. Porter. London: Routledge. p. 51.
12. Freud, S. (2003). The Uncanny. London: Penguin.
13. Baum, F. L. (1989) *Ozma of Oz*. New York. William Morrow.
14. Čapek, K. (2004) R.U.R. London. Penguin.
15. Bladerunner.
16. Ex Machina.
17. While many take the origami unicorn as an unambiguous confirmation of Deckard's replicant status, it remains only a forceful hint.
18. Bladerunner.
19. Meillassoux, Q. (2008) *After Finitude: An Essay on the Necessity of Contingency*. London. Continuum. p. 26.
20. Ibid.
21. Braidotti, R. (2013) *The Posthuman*. London. Polity Press. p. 189.
22. Hook, D. (2017) *Six Moments in Lacan: An Introduction*. London. Routledge.
23. Lacan, J. (2006) 'The Mirror Stage as Formative of the *I* Function as Revealed in Psychoanalytic Experience' in Lacan, J. (2006) *Écrits: The First* Complete Edition in English, trans. B. Fink. London: Norton. pp. 75–81.
24. Husserl, E. (1991) Cartesian Meditations: An Introduction to Phenomenology, trans. D. Cairns. London: Kluwer Academic Publishers.
25. Lacan, J. (1977/1960), 'Subversion of the Subject and Dialectic of Desire' in Lacan, J. (2006) *Écrits: The First* Complete Edition in English, trans. B. Fink. London: Norton. p. 694.
26. Lacan, J. (2016) *The Sinthome: The Seminar of Jacques Lacan, Book XXIII*. London. Polity Press.
27. Braidotti, R. (2013) *The Posthuman*. London. Polity Press. p. 189.
28. Dick, P.K. (1996) *Do Androids Dream of Electric Sheep*? New York. Del Rey.

Bibliography

Baum, F.L. 1989. *Ozma of Oz*. New York: William Morrow.
Braidotti, R. 2013. *The Posthuman*. London: Polity Press.
Čapek, K. 2004. *R.U.R.* London: Penguin.
Descartes, R. 2014. *Meditations on First Philosophy*. Cambridge: Cambridge University Press.
Dick, P.K. 1996. *Do Androids Dream of Electric Sheep?* New York: Del Rey.
Freud, S. 1966. A Project for a Scientific Psychology. In *The Complete Works of Sigmund Freud, Vol. 1: Pre-psychoanalytical Publications and Unpublished Drafts*. Trans. J. Strachey. London: Hogarth.
———. 2003. *The Uncanny*. London: Penguin.
Hegel, G.W.F. 1967. *The Phenomenology of Mind*. Trans. J. B. Baillie. New York: Harper and Row.
Hook, D. 2017. *Six Moments in Lacan: An Introduction*. London: Routledge.
Husserl, E. 1991. *Cartesian Meditations: An Introduction to Phenomenology*. Trans. D. Cairns. London: Kluwer Academic Publishers.
Lacan, J. 1977/1973. *The Seminar of Jacques Lacan, Book XI: The Four Fundamental Concepts of Psychoanalysis*. Trans. A. Sheridan. London: Penguin.
———. 1992. *The Seminar of Jacques Lacan, Book VII: The Ethics of Psychoanalysis (1959–1960)*. Trans. D. Porter. London: Routledge.
———. 1998. *Séminaire, Tome 4 : la Relation d'Objet*. Paris: Seuil.
———. 2006a. Subversion of the Subject and Dialectic of Desire. In *Écrits: The First Complete Edition*. Trans. B. Fink. London: W. W. Norton.
———. 2006b. The Mirror Stage as Formative of the *I* Function as Revealed in Psychoanalytic Experience. In *Écrits: The First Complete Edition*. Trans. B. Fink. London: W. W. Norton.
———. 2016. *The Seminar of Jacques Lacan, Book XXIII: The Sinthome*. London: Polity Press.
Meillassoux, Q. 2008. *After Finitude: An Essay on the Necessity of Contingency*. London: Continuum.
Metzinger, T. 2003. *Being No One: The Self-Model Theory of Subjectivity*. Cambridge, MA: MIT Press.
Nietzsche, F. 2001. *Beyond Good and Evil*. Trans. J. Norman. Cambridge: Cambridge University Press.

ASMR Mania, Trigger-Chasing, and the Anxiety of Digital Repletion

Hugh S. Manon

To the uninitiated, YouTube autonomous sensory meridian response (ASMR) videos are either pleasurably or painfully excessive. The videos' performers—who customarily refer to themselves as 'ASMRtists'—speak directly into the camera, very close, in sibilant whispers, consonant repetitions, and with an attitude of oversolicitous caregiving. The goal of such speech often is explicitly stated by the speaker: to elicit tingling sensations in the beholder's head, neck, and spine. This response has been described as a kind of nonsexual 'head orgasm,' and devotees of ASMR return to the videos in order to reactivate the sensation. Common ASMR scenarios include enactments of 'the kind of close personal attention you get when someone cuts your hair, certain sounds like tapping or brushing, and perhaps most bizarrely of all, observing someone doing something trivial very carefully and diligently.'[1]

The discourse around and within ASMR videos stresses that tingles are elusive, precarious, and subject to failure—experienced to varying

H.S. Manon (✉)
Clark University, Worcester, MA, USA

G. Basu Thakur, J.M. Dickstein (eds.), *Lacan and the Nonhuman*,
The Palgrave Lacan Series, DOI 10.1007/978-3-319-63817-1_12

degrees, and by some individuals but not others. For those not susceptible, the effect can be the opposite of pleasure: a mildly annoying or intensely repulsive misophonia. Understood from a Lacanian perspective, these two qualities of ASMR—its evanescence and its propensity to produce both pleasure and pain—help one to situate users at a nexus of desire, drive, and anxiety. It is exactly in these terms that this chapter rethinks this emergent millennial media phenomenon. By encouraging its users to desire drive itself—to seek an encounter with the pulsating, automatized, mechanical forces that make desire cyclical and, ultimately, unsatisfiable—ASMR confronts them with the nonhuman forces that undergird their own sense of being, while at the same time providing a respite from contemporary forms of anxiety.

ASMR creators and enthusiasts persistently articulate their desire for repeatable and consistent tingles around the word 'trigger.' In proceeding to probe this term, a contrarian stance is taken here; that is, despite their doting qualities and widely variable approaches, ASMR videos do not desire to fulfill a lack. Instead, ASMR trigger-chasing must be understood as symptomatic of broader digital–millennial trends in its repudiation of the *lack of lack itself*, which Lacan identifies as 'anxiety.' ASMR videos exist in a context in which the trusted reliability and lossless plenitude of digital technology have become problems in themselves. In pointed ways, digital culture lacks the lack on which desire is founded: It delivers too much, too quickly, too easily, and too dependably.

In this context of media overflow, ASMR offers a reprieve by temporarily transforming the beholder into a nonhuman object whose lack is absolute, whose desire for connectedness fails, and whose experience is fixedly partial. By objectifying the viewer-as-subject, ASMR mobilizes the insular, pulsatile, blindly circular trajectory of the drive against human desire's troublesome propensity to exceed its goals and to lapse into anxiety.

As such, ASMR's emphasis on pseudo-interactivity directly impacts the videos' content, which typically does not involve staging encounters with lovers or actual maternal/paternal caregivers, but instead with opticians, barbers, salespeople, suit-fitters, and other functionaries whose attentiveness is rote. In ASMR videos, we behold neither a genuinely caring caregiver, nor an uncaring or sadistic disciplinarian but rather an indifferent drone—a waxwork contraption that appears where the loving mother ought to be. It is this rendezvous with a nonhuman pseudo-partner, not connectivity or caregiving per se, that the anxious millennial subject covertly longs for—that is, seeking a connection with disconnection itself in the form of excessively proximate sounds and mechanical, objectifying verbal patter. When ASMR succeeds, the beholder is not physically or emotionally satisfied, but instead is 'triggered' at the level of drive, like a binary switch or sensor. At this moment of release, one physically senses desire being unseated by drive, as the subject assumes the status of a nonhuman object.

By the mid-2010s, YouTube and Reddit had become the primary social media platforms on which ASMR videos were exchanged and discussed. As a most basic form of discernment, online fans made (and continue to make) a critical distinction between two broad types of ASMR video productions. The first type is the intentional or 'roleplay' video, in which a performer enacts a fictional service-providing scenario, usually with the viewer occupying the customer's point of view. The second type is the 'unintentional' ASMR video, often flagged as such in a subject header, in which a real-world interaction has been captured and uploaded, and then subsequently discovered by ASMR users who misappropriate the video for its tingle-triggering properties. The sections that follow focus in turn on these two types of video, and the two dominant aesthetics they embody, respectively: whispered consonance and rote patter. By correlating these aspects—both of which evacuate meaning in order to foreground noise—we can come to some conclusions about the millennial subject's fascination with trigger-chasing; the relationship between desire, drive, and anxiety; and the new and fairly unique anxieties facing digital natives.

Hear Hear: The Aesthetics of Proximity

A remarkable feature of ASMR videos is that their tingle-inducing stimuli tend to emerge in scenarios that are palpably native, commonplace, *heimliche*. The background for the ASMR trigger is not itself extreme or excessive; it is subtle, calm, and unobtrusive. Against this normalized backdrop, low-amplitude sounds, which would otherwise be indiscernible in their softness, rise to the surface, arresting the viewer's attention through extreme close-up shots and microphonic amplification. In this way, ASMR videos aim to evoke a sense of *loud quietness*, or *sharp softness*, resulting in tingles. No drugs are ingested to produce this effect, nor does the beholder need to chant a mantra. No vibrators, gravity boots, carnival rides, or other apparatuses are required for tingles to occur. On the contrary, when ASMR is triggered, the trigger must pointedly come from the mundane.

Although none of the experiential categories (e.g., doppelgangers, injuries to the eye, random numbers reoccurring, etc.) enumerated by Freud in his 1919 essay, 'The Uncanny,' strictly concur with ASMR's trigger effect, the fact that a quotidian event involuntarily causes one's scalp and neck to tingle surely does approximate the homey setting in which the *unheimliche* suddenly appears. By turning banal discourse on its head through amplification and sheer repetition, ASMR instantiates Freud's claim that 'the uncanny' involves 'uncover[ing]…secret forces,' but does so via a kind of neurological hot-wiring of the subject's body.[2]

When ASMR is triggered, there is a sense that one's neural pathways are being haunted by their own proto-human evolutionary vestiges; that the pleasure of the infant, or the cave-dweller, or the social-grooming primate has reignited within the millennial adult-human's sensorum, of its own accord and with real physical/corporeal effects. ASMR is always noted as being pleasurable by those who experience it, whereas those who do not experience it often find the videos painful (e.g., misophonic or offensive in other ways) to endure. This dichotomy raises the question: *Is it possible to have a pleasurable uncanny experience?* Because ASMR seems to be just that.

To explore this connection between ASMR and the Freudian uncanny—and consequently the relationship between Lacan's conceptions of desire, drive, and anxiety—it will be helpful to outline some characteristic ASMR scenarios, techniques, and structures. Perhaps most obviously, ASMR videos involve a relation of proximity between speaker and beholder. Like anxiety itself, which Roberto Harari describes as a 'border or edge phenomenon' between desire and *jouissance*,[3] ASMR's *mise-en-scène* of proximity exists on the knife-edge between 'not enough' and 'too much.' The beholder is constantly aware that the ASMRtist is situated either right up against the camera, right up against the microphone, or poised to occupy these positions in a forthcoming shot. Space and sound become inextricable, as the extreme close-up of the performer's face becomes a metonymy for the amplification and excess detail a microphone affords.

A primary question, then, concerns why ASMR is so uniformly dedicated to scenarios of proximity, not some other audiovisual arrangement. The answer can be found in a second feature that is so obvious that, to my knowledge, no one has ever taken the time to note it. That is, the source of the words and sounds we hear in ASMR videos must invariably emit from a *singular* body. In any given video, whether intentional or unintentional, one single person does the talking, folding, unwrapping, or tapping, and so on, and the focus remains squarely on her or him. The very rare (always flagged as 'special') occurrences of dual-presenter or alternating 'tag team' ASMR videos only reaffirm this rule of singularity.

Moreover, in unintentional videos in which two people are necessarily present on camera (e.g., in medical exams, barbershop shaves, massages, etc.), most of the action and talking is conducted by a single person of authority, whereas the 'customer' in the exchange remains inert and semisilent. Correspondingly, on the receiving side of an ASMR video, there is only ever a singular viewer, not a group; this is something that the discourse of all ASMRtists tacitly acknowledges, all the time. Why is this? The answer has to do with the uncanny borderline status of *proximate objects*, an ambiguous phrase that bespeaks neither an obvious absolute lack on the part of the subject, nor a fully satisfying attainment.

ASMR's fundamental approach is to repeatedly stage a focused, one-on-one binary in which a series of sonic objects are successively reviewed, very closely, right on the spatial perimeter that distinguishes human subject from nonhuman object. Such tight, binary arrangements necessarily confuse the divisions between here and there, this and that, interior and exterior. In this way, the videos divide their audience into two groups: drive-seekers, who may find bodily enjoyment in ASMR sounds; and desire-seekers, who will experience a suffocating anxiety, and wish they could close their ears.

As psychoanalysis insists, there is a deceptively stark difference between nearness and actual arrival. ASMR's approach to sound lays bare the idea that these two states (i.e., closeness and presence), which are usually conceived as synonymous, are in fact categorical opposites. For viewers who 'get' ASMR, the videos' staging of aural proximity is self-evidently not a full arrival, with the visual barrier imposed by the screen denying the very sorts of haptic connection that the videos' soundtracks consistently foreground. This ever-present lack, or gap, in the process of attainment is what lends ASMR an alleged therapeutic value that is frequently touted by both users and content-producers.

ASMR videos only seem to stage a kind of perfectly caring satisfaction; they only seem to provide a consistently accessible mother-figure at the click of a link. In place of these satisfactions, ASMR instead delivers a constant reminder of its own status as ersatz attainment, and this distanced falseness is exactly what the ASMR community craves. Although ASMR users and content providers likely will disagree with such an antihumanist assessment, Lacanian theory makes clear that ASMR trigger-chasing involves a willful commitment to go nowhere—an engagement not with desire, but with the drive, the goals of which are nonobvious and the pleasures of which are quite literally pointless in human terms.

In the words of Lacanian theorist Mladen Dolar, whose 2006 book, *A Voice and Nothing More*, compellingly informs this chapter: '[T]he voice stands at a paradoxical and ambiguous topological spot, at the intersection of language and the body, but this intersection belongs to neither.'[4] Accordingly, ASMR is not an interaction that aims at intimacy, but instead is a transaction driven by what Lacan calls 'extimacy'—an 'internal externality,' an 'expropriated intimacy.'[5] ASMR's approach to audio reminds one, sometimes painfully, that speech and voice are not the same, and that the voice is an object of the drive.

For Lacan, two factors place the voice on the side of the object, rather than on the side of the subject. First, the voice is a supplement of the body, extending outward from it; and second, the voice is a marker of 'the division into an exterior and an interior,' while not belonging to either.[6] This bodily margin is constitutive for the subject because it is here that lack most obviously materializes. Substances appearing at or around the body's various rim-like orifices—borderline objects that appear partially without and partially within—comprise what Lacan calls *objets petits a*.

Like the other objects of the drive (e.g., the breast, the feces, the gaze), the voice occupies the 'zone of overlapping, the crossing, the extimate'[7]; in addition, Dolar is careful to note that the word 'extimate' is 'the excellent Lacanian word for the uncanny.'[8] It is precisely in such a space that ASMR appears as a series of pleasurably uncanny sonic objects—music for non-humans, as it were.

A staple element of ASMR roleplay videos, and the one that initially allowed them to be identified as a distinct Internet phenomena, is whispering—a hyperproximate mode of speech that serves as an optimal carrier for what is hereafter called the 'object-voice.' In videos by successful YouTube ASMRtists, such as 'TheWaterwhispers,' 'WhispersRed,' and 'Heather Feather,' the soundtrack is dominated by barely phonated whispers and exceedingly gentle talking, the point of which is not to promote actual inaudibility. Rather, whispering conveys a sense of abstraction through proximity, with the microphone greatly amplifying the contours of speech. Nothing is being confided except for the hushed tonalities of confidence itself, and the excessive closeness makes one all but forget what is being said, which is suitably hollow and often patently arbitrary. Like cool drops of water landing on a hot skillet, the consonance and sibilance of ASMR whispering materializes the evaporation of meaning at the boundary between subject and object; in the case of audition, the rims of the ears themselves.

As of August 2017, with more than 18 million views, the most-viewed ASMR roleplay video on YouTube is entitled '*_* Oh such a good 3D-sound ASMR video *_*' by ASMRtist GentleWhispering, a Russian émigré to the United States named Maria who speaks English with a thick accent.[9] As many ASMR videos do, it utilizes a stereophonic microphone arrangement, placed out of sight very near the camera, to approximate a '3-D' effect when played back on headphones. As Maria fondles and taps on a stiff-bristled hairbrush, her dialogue is entirely descriptive and banal—a delivery mechanism for her whispers, but not primarily a carrier of meaning:

> I truly enjoy the sound of it when you run your fingers over it—over the bristles. It actually feels nice, as well as sounds nice. [Pause in speech; scratching and tapping sounds are prominent.] And if you can tap right on

> the edge, just slightly, it sounds [long pause] quite relaxing. So I could do that from here [moves brush off-screen right; scratching sounds], on one side for you, and then do the same on the other side [moves brush off-screen left; tapping and scratching sounds continue]—run my fingers through the bristles—and that gentle tapping, that will feel really good. The tapping sounds remind me of the sound of the rain.

If this transcription of Maria's words reads like rudimentary, prattling nonsense, this is entirely the point. The pleasure of ASMR crystallizes when sounds eclipse meaning, when the speaker's discourse is reduced to babbling noncommunication, a pure pretense. What the general viewer cannot fail to notice in such discourse, and what the ASMR devotee actively seeks, is an encounter with the 'object-voice.'

According to Dolar, the object-voice in Lacanian terms is 'the material element recalcitrant to meaning,' 'the extralingual element which enables speech phenomena, but cannot itself be discerned by linguistics.'[10] The object-voice manifests not in the production of meaning but in the idiosyncratic sounds that convey it—'the accent, the intonation, and the timbre.'[11] In other words, in ASMR, we are not hearing words or meaning, but instead *hearing hearing* itself in the form of the object-voice. A fascinating corollary to this is the conundrum of what it would mean for the ears to look rather than hear. Given the videos' heavy emphasis on sounds of tactility, clicky resistance, and abrasion, what is ASMR if not the subject reading with one's ears? To do so results in a nullification of meaningful speech, and a correspondingly blunt reaffirmation of the indifference and inertia of the voice in its pure form, as an object of the drive.[12]

To pursue an object of desire involves a conscious recognition of one's goal, and a movement toward it; to seek ASMR tingles entails a more precarious, arguably nonhuman pursuit in which one confronts the unconscious directly, by seeking out pleasures that are oblique, tangential, and strange. In psychoanalytic parlance, the word 'drive' is not usually employed as an active verb; however, if it were, we could more easily recognize ASMR as a 'desire to drive,' or better yet, a subcultural tactic in which users and content-providers cooperate in an attempt to drive (over) desire.

Renata Salecl explains that '[d]rive and desire each have a different relation to the symbolic structure':

> Desire is essentially linked to the law, since it always searches for something that is prohibited or unavailable. The logic of desire would be: 'It is prohibited to do this, but I will nonetheless do it.' Drive, in contrast, does not care about prohibition: it is not concerned about overcoming the law. Drive's logic is: 'I do not want to do this, but I am nonetheless doing it.' Thus, we have a contrary logic in drive since the subject does *not* desire to do something, but nonetheless enjoys doing exactly that.[13]

We know that the whispered speech of the ASMRtist is triggering an enjoyment of the drive because we sense a palpably 'off' quality in the experience; these sounds should not be producing pleasure but are doing so nonetheless. In Lee Edelman's helpful formulation: We know the drive is at play because 'we experience our enjoyment despite ourselves.'[14] The vibratory head-and-neck buzz enjoyed by ASMR users is a signal that this goal of engaging the drive has been attained, and correspondingly that desire's fundamental crisis-point (i.e., the absence of lack itself that Lacan identifies as anxiety) has been quelled, put on pause.

Having defined the most basic ASMR aesthetic, proximate whispering, as an instantiation of the Lacanian voice as *objet petit a*—as well as a site of drive-based pleasure for those who partake—the following section addresses the ways in which the disinterestedness of a speaker, exemplified in a celebrated 'unintentional' ASMR video, contributes to a radical objectification of the ASMR viewer. In doing so, it also provides a second opportunity for the subject to drive (over) desire, and thus find temporary relief from millennial forms of anxiety.

Lip Service: Desubjectifying the Subject

In his essay 'The Uncanny,' Freud notes that children are 'especially fond of treating their dolls as if they were alive,' which can lead to certain uncanny effects.[15] ASMR is a reverse arrangement in which real people have the uncanny sense that they are being treated like dolls; or, more specifically, like children treat dolls: by combing their hair, speaking quietly to them, and devoting excessive care to what is obviously a nonhuman toy. Indeed, much ASMR content is centered on this keyword 'care'—caregiving, taking care, carefulness, and so on. Nonetheless, the crucial conceptual leap, and the one that the limited existing scholarship on ASMR fails to make, is that ASMR care is most always *care for an object,* even when that object is a human subject (i.e., the viewer and/or listener).

In ASMR, the beholder's own body is treated as a passive sensor, bristling reflexively to certain stimuli, the same as a Venus flytrap responds to the landing of an insect. In such moments, the subject is conferred with object status—not loved but instead groomed, maintained, serviced. In turn, ASMR devotees come to relish, and not avoid, their own capacity for nonhuman reactivity, celebrating the Freudian subject's uncanny sense that there exist 'automatic—mechanical—processes [...] hidden beneath the familiar image of a living person.'[16]

Outsiders not familiar with ASMR's modus operandi almost invariably view the YouTube genre as a thinly veiled exercise in on-demand maternal care, a supposition that the predominance of female ASMRtists does not repudiate. For example, in a 2014 *today.com* article, a journalist makes the following observation:

> People might associate these triggers with pleasant experiences. That whispering might remind someone of mom lulling her to sleep. A haircut might spark fond memories of Saturdays spent with dad at the barbershop.[17]

Such commentary misses the mark by failing to discern that ASMR is ontologically noninteractive, foregrounding not care and attentiveness, but its blockage. Everything the ASMRtist says and does is fundamentally a form of disinterested prattle, and although the trope of the solicitously concerned maternal figure enables the genre, it is ancillary to its effects.

ASMR discourse is nothing at all like the personalized, adaptive attention of the sensual voice of Samantha (Scarlett Johansson), the computer operating system in Spike Jonze's 2013 film *Her*, that responds in new and different ways with each passing interaction. The problem with Samantha is not that she is nonhuman, but that her artificial intelligence has developed to the point of being *too* human. In contrast to Samantha's free-flowing, truly dialogic interactivity, which she learns through practice, the ASMR voice optimally addresses its beholder in an all-too-slick sales pitch that betrays endless prior rehearsal, an inflexible preordained agenda, and an overall lack of humanistic concern.

In a 2013 GentleWhispering video called '~•••~Relaxing Physical Therapist Visit~•••~,' Maria tellingly portrays both a deskbound office receptionist and the physical therapist herself, never acknowledging any difference or point of transition between these mutually exclusive forms of employment.[18] The reason for this strained continuity is that, for ASMR's purposes, all caregiving personnel are identical by virtue of their ability to objectify their customer. When, early on, receptionist Maria says, 'I'm sorry about the accident. … I hope you're feeling better,' she delivers these words in a rote, phony manner that suggests that the words are part of a quasi-scripted routine she goes through with all patients.

It is not actual consistent care that ASMR aims to produce, but instead a self-evidently artificial going-through-the-motions of what care is supposed to look and sound like. Virtually any scenario in which a speaker might go through the motions can be a potential ASMR trigger site, with the caregiver's empathic stance relegated to little more than a coatrack on which to hang the empty, objectifying patter of the drive.

According to the *Oxford English Dictionary*, the noun 'patter' means two distinct things, both relevant to ASMR. Patter is 'a rapid succession of light taps, or similar slight sounds'[19]—an effect that is the central subject of hundreds of ASMR videos—and also 'smooth, persuasive talk; especially the rapid speech used by a street trader, salesperson, etc., to attract or cajole customers.'[20] The second meaning of 'patter' etymologically derives from Catholic prayer rituals, specifically 'from the rapid and mechanical way in which the paternoster was often repeated, e.g. in the rosary.'[21] The crucial element here is that in a salesman's patter, as in the 'paternoster' recited by churchgoers, the materiality of speech tends to obscure the signifying content of the words, rendering the speaker's discourse strangely nonhuman, and thus (under non-ASMR circumstances) worthy of skepticism or disdain. In patter, we are more aware of the sound of what is being said than we are of the meaning; more aware of the delivery mechanism than the goods being served.[22]

The rote, patter-driven aspect of ASMR is best exemplified in the second major category of videos, known by users as 'unintentional ASMR.'[23] A cornerstone in the conceptual development of unintentional ASMR is the North American public television program, *The Joy of Painting* (1983–1994), hosted by calm-talking landscape painter Bob Ross. Although Ross clearly operates with teacherly intent, viewers are free to siphon off some surplus enjoyment from the gentle deliberateness of his voice and his methodical application of paints using brushes and palette knives. All unintentional ASMR is premised on such misappropriations of real-world source material.

One of the most celebrated unintentional ASMR videos on YouTube is entitled 'Cranial Nerve Test with Pat LaFontaine & Dr. James Kelly.'[24] Taped in 1998, the video presents an extensive, noninvasive nerve exam, with lots of bodily and facial touching, along with many questions and answers between doctor and patient.[25] The doctor in charge is clearly a skilled neurologist, and the subject of the examination is a well-known professional hockey player whose career on the ice was ended by a series of concussions; they are the only people on screen in a typically bland examination room. The video is professionally recorded with a tripod-mounted camcorder and microphone boom (sometimes visible), and its nine-plus minutes unfold in a standard, third-person medium shot. The office is quiet and the two men are rarely more than four feet apart, permitting much of the doctor's dialogue to be spoken in hushed, calm tones.

The video is part of a series sponsored by BrainLine.org, 'a national multimedia project offering information and resources about preventing, treating, and living with TBI [traumatic brain injury],'[26] and it is easy to imagine that it has served well its intended purpose of educating people affected by traumatic brain injury regarding what to expect during such an exam. Still, knowing that the video's high view count (more than 3.3 million at the time of this chapter's writing) is largely the result of the video being exploited for unintended tingles can help to clarify its trigger points. It is easy to imagine, for instance, that ASMR-susceptible viewers experience shivers at the point when Dr. Kelly speaks softly—in an almost voiceless consonant whisper—the words 'okay, good,' affirming that LaFontaine has responded normally to a test of his peripheral vision and that the exam will proceed. There are a total of 12 instances of 'okay, good' in the nine-minute video, all spoken in this manner.

Similarly, viewers may be triggered by the subtle, but entirely audible rubbing of Dr. Kelly's sleeve against the body of his wool suit during the strength-testing portions of the exam, or by the crinkling of the sanitary paper that lines the examination table. As Rob Gallagher notes in his outstanding essay on ASMR aesthetics, such noises are forms of what Michel Chion calls 'materializing sound indices' (MSI); that is, they render a kind of primordial, felt sense of the object producing the sound.[27]

Most distinctive however—and much remarked about in the YouTube video's comments section—are the points during the examination when Dr. Kelly engages in a benign doctorly patter, clearly developed over many years of administering such exams. In his well-rehearsed examination procedure, one element follows very quickly after another, with each new exercise and command delivered calmly and dispassionately. At one point early on, Dr. Kelly instructs LaFontaine to 'close [his] eyes real tight—real tight, like you got soap in 'em.' The doctor presses his thumbs onto LaFontaine's eyebrows, forcing them upward. 'Don't let me open 'em up,' he says, followed by a quickly enunciated 'fight fight fight fight fight.' This unexpected command to 'fight' makes sense when we consider Kelly's work with athletes and combat veterans.

In the context of the exceptionally civilized and nonviolent exchange between the two men, the word 'fight' becomes an ASMR trigger precisely because its idiosyncratic phrasing belies repeated past use. All such patients, one assumes, are told by Dr. Kelly to 'fight fight fight fight fight'; it is easy to see that there is nothing genuinely personal in this apparently personal touch. The fact that Pat LaFontaine is a real individual, with real past medical problems specific to him (i.e., the now-resolved facial paralysis noted by both), only underscores the fact that Dr. Kelly is for all purposes disengaged, dispassionate, and 'clinical' in the most literal sense. He certainly appears attentive, intelligent, and kind, but even these attributes are a strategic part of his bedside manner, and thus somewhat false.

The difference between patter and speech finds its somatic equivalent in the difference between the word 'touch' (something a caregiver, friend, or lover does to a partner) and the word 'palpate' (something a doctor does to a patient). The content of ASMR videos does not involve touching, which in real life may be employed to produce various forms of pleasure, but instead *palpation*, which by definition is indifferent to the production of pleasure. The source of ASMR tingles resides precisely in this monodirectional indifference. Something is being done *to* us, rather than *for* us.

By way of contrast, consider how alarming it would be if a hair stylist, a suit-fitter, or a door-to-door salesperson cared too much about their client—touching rather than palpating—thus crossing the line of social propriety. ASMR videos do not take liberties in this way; they are the furthest thing possible from the representation of desire one witnesses in 1970s pornography, the dominant trope of which involves a doctor, a plumber, or a pizza delivery person violating cultural taboos by engaging in sex acts with a patron. At once rejecting and offering an alternative to such straightforward acts of desire, ASMR appears at first glance to move in the direction of desire's consummation; however, very quickly it stops short, fetishizing the 'customer experience'—a memorized and rehearsed, mock form of care with entirely nonromantic, vaguely apathetic connotations. In this way, ASMR videos only pretend to deliver the staging and satisfaction of a desire, making clear through rote patter that the viewer is (or should be) watching solely for the drive.

YouTube is the ASMR format par excellence. To my knowledge, there are no real-life ASMR clubs featuring hands-on interaction, nor are there pay-to-play, webcam-based live ASMR sessions. There is a good reason for this. Were an ASMRtist to perform routines interactively, or in the presence of a real-life subject, the performer would likely respond in a personalized way to the subject's responses and would be less able to continue in a manner that is rehearsed, rote, dispassionate, and thus effective in nonhuman terms. Any truly interactive form of an ASMRtist's roleplay would subjectify the subject rather than objectifying the individual, thus nullifying one of ASMR's primary tingle-inducing vectors.

To be clear, ASMR can and does appear in certain real-life situations, but when it does, it emerges in accidental and tangential ways. A Reddit user, known as 'AwsumSaus,' reveals a telling example of how ASMR's subject-objectifying tingles can develop vis-à-vis one's daily work routines:

> I honestly don't watch ASMR for the relaxation, I watch it for the tingles. These will never beat the real-life tingles I get, for example while watching someone interact with something of mine (it's weird, but when people used to browse the section I 'owned' at work = tingles).[28]

To clarify, the user is describing a former retail sales position, in which certain employees were responsible for maintaining individual sections of a large store. Her tingles were the result of individual customers entering her quasi-proprietary retail territory, her 'section.' The word 'owned' here denotes a quasi-anthropomorphic link, felt by many in retail, that they function as a part of the store-as-body and are somehow indistinguishable from it.

In the cited example, ASMR tingles result not from a personal interaction between worker and customer, but from the staff member 'watching' the customer perusing a well-maintained 'owned' area, one in which the border between subject (the retail clerk) and object (the store and its merchandise) has been blurred. The meticulously straightened and carefully organized items for sale are both 'something of mine' and decidedly someone else's (i.e., the property of the corporation that owns the store). The clerk's tingles result from the sense that she is physically jacked-in to the store-as-object—a kind of nonhuman extension or appendage of it—and that the customers are perusing her own (inert, passively displayed) body, as much as they are perusing the objects for sale.

Similar effects reportedly have been triggered by medical magnetic resonance imaging (MRI) scans, by automatic car washes, and by getting an oil change at a facility where the driver remains in the vehicle.[29] In such real-world circumstances, as in unintentional videos, ASMR pleasure is the result of an 'uncanny' collision between subjectification and objectification, humanity and the nonhuman; tingles are a sign that one is presently occupying both states at once, vibrating rapidly between them in an oscillation that purposefully goes nowhere.

Conclusion: Driving Away Digital Anxiety

As someone who does not experience ASMR, I must confess that I have never understood, never *felt*, any validity in users' constant refrains about ASMR's therapeutic value for sufferers of anxiety, insomnia, depression, and migraines. How could a tingly head-buzz possibly eradicate or assuage such problems? Nevertheless, if ASMR engages subjects in the way suggested here—not at the level of desire, which is the trajectory on which anxiety develops, but at the level of drive—then it accords that ASMR's drive-focused enjoyment could temporarily excuse the subject from experiencing anxiety in desire's terms, as a lack of lack itself.

In *The Ticklish Subject*, Slavoj Žižek argues that drive is presubjective, head-less, a kind of nonhuman 'acephalous force which persists in its repetitive movement' and thus involves neither a goal that can be pursued, nor a sense of anxiety after reaching that goal.[30] This, however, leaves the question: Can drive itself be pursued? Or more precisely: Can subjects strategically put themselves in a position where drive might tend to emerge? ASMR, I conclude, is a quintessential example of such active drive-seeking, a fact that becomes clear when we view ASMR's peculiar practices both within and against a backdrop of excessive digital connectedness.

To make sense of contemporary modes of anxiety, and of ASMR's purported therapeutic value, one final question is posed: What has happened to desire-inspiring prohibition in the era of digital transmission? Certainly, the potential for technology-fueled interactivity has vastly increased during the twenty-first century, and I want to claim that rather than increasing our enjoyment in turn, digital technology exposes users to a tyranny of connectedness, instantaneity, and perfectibility—three qualities that sound like laudable attributes, but that ultimately serve as the platform on which an anxiety-inspiring acklessness takes shape.

In the era of the digital, the spatiotemporal delays built into past communication technologies have been eradicated. Letters are delivered in microseconds, not days or weeks. Images arrive instantaneously from around the world, and in vibrant high-definition color. Perfect copies are derived from other perfect copies without loss of clarity. Two-way audio conversation is possible in unprecedentedly remote locales. 'Selfies' are viewed on screen as they are taken, optimally framed, with mistakes deleted instantly and filters applied, to arrive at a perfect image of oneself to send to friends. Perhaps most significantly, all technology has become affordably 'in reach' for average consumers.

Having a high-definition, web-integrated video camera in one's pocket imbues daily life with an expectation of unfailing connectedness rather than intermittence, isolation, and lack. In all these ways, Lacan's dictum that 'anxiety isn't the signal of a lack, but [...] the failing of the support that lack provides' returns with a vengeance.[31] In this context of digital suffusion and the excessive perfectibility of millennial media forms, ASMR is a hallmark counterpractice wherein the subject short-circuits desire by demanding *jouissance* directly, thus circumventing any necessity for prohibition as a support and nullifying the anxiety that comes with too much attainment.

Enabled by digital transcoding, fiber-optic networks, and high-speed processing, the millennial subject's developing investments in trigger-chasing exist precisely as a drive-based, anxiety-busting response to the oversaturation of digital culture itself, including social media's injunction that no one should ever 'miss out' on what is happening in her or his absence. In the context of free-flowing, digitally catalyzed interactivity between subjects, ASMR purveys the opposite: a belabored, mechanized, one-way transaction in which the viewer is acted on but not active. Whereas any such objectification of the beholder would seem at first glance to *create* anxiety by reducing the subject to something less than human, on the contrary, the drive-based pursuit engendered by ASMR works to upend anxiety by remaining indifferent to prohibition's role in the dialectic of desire.

In the words of Jacques-Alain Miller: 'The drive couldn't care less about prohibition; it knows nothing of prohibition and certainly doesn't dream of transgressing it. The drive follows its own bent and always obtains satisfaction.'[32] In being triggered, or even in having toyed with the idea that triggers exist, we are instantaneously mobilized not as humanistic Cartesian subjects consciously pursuing enjoyment, but as nonhuman objects that instantaneously have it or do not, as the case may be. In such an arrangement, there is no obstacle to surmount, and thus never any question of anxiety beyond attainment. There is only the capricious, all-at-once buzzing of *jouissance*.

Both as an aesthetic and a practice, ASMR is emblematically millennial. Regardless of whether culture is broadly aware of ASMR's existence, it is certainly on the rise, and for those who partake, it is a definitive marker of twenty-first century living. Nevertheless, in the final analysis, it is perhaps the 'not for everyone' aspect of ASMR that is ontologically definitive, precisely because the evanescence and inconsistency of ASMR's trigger-culture cuts directly against digital technology's hegemonic aims. Facebook works for everyone. Netflix works for everyone. Smartphones work for everyone. On the contrary, however, ASMR only works for a limited few. Individual videos (and parts of videos) trigger certain individuals but not others, for reasons no one can fully explain.

Functioning for many as a do-it-yourself form of therapy, ASMR is not a matter of regularizing or standardizing triggers. Rather, the point of the genre is to perpetuate the notion that some triggers work for some people and not others. As Rob Gallagher notes: 'In [Reddit] forums like r/asmr, questions of provenance, content, meaning and intention are irrelevant. Debates over symbolism, subtext and irony are abandoned. Only one question matters: does it trigger you or not?'[33] The seeming impossibility of unifying around a singular 'master trigger' is exactly what makes a trigger a trigger: *We mostly do not agree* because we mostly do not respond to ASMR in the same way.

Indeed, it would be correct to say that ASMR 'works' even for viewers who have never felt any tingles. What is pleasurable is not the tingles themselves, but the fact that they cannot be pursued along the well-trodden paths of desire. Appearing in the border-zone between subject and object, human and nonhuman, the pleasure of ASMR triggers are unspeakable, as all pleasures of the drive must be. It remains to be seen how new technologies, such as virtual reality headsets, will reorient ASMR's subject-objectifying practices, as well as to what extent ASMR's drive-focused subculture might speak to mainstream audiences.

Notes

1. Hannah Maslen and Rebecca Roache, 'ASMR and Absurdity,' *Practical Ethics* (blog), University of Oxford, July 29, 2015, http://blog.practicalethics.ox.ac.uk/2015/07/asmr-and-absurdity/
2. Sigmund Freud, *The Uncanny*, trans. David McLintock (New York: Penguin, 2003), p. 150.

3. Roberto Harari, *Lacan's Seminar on Anxiety: An Introduction*, trans. Jane C. Lamb-Ruiz (New York: Other Press, 2001), p. 36.
4. Of concern in the drive are precisely such border-like bodily rims: not the stomach that digests food, but the lips and teeth; not the ear canal and eardrum that registers sound, but the external auricle and the void it surrounds. Mladen Dolar, *A Voice and Nothing More* (Cambridge: MIT Press, 2006), p. 73.
5. Ibid., p. 96.
6. Ibid., p. 81.
7. Ibid.
8. Ibid., p. 96.
9. '*_* Oh Such a Good 3D-Sound ASMR Video *_*,' *YouTube.com*, last modified September 7, 2012, https://www.youtube.com/watch?v=RVpfHgC3ye0
10. Dolar (2006), p. 15.
11. Ibid., p. 20.
12. Michael Connor makes a similar claim about ASMR's tendency to substitute one sense for another: '[W]atching ASMR videos of people folding towels is more pleasurable for many people than the real act of folding towels. It's almost like what is satisfying about them is not the tactile sensation itself, but the fact that this tactile sensation is triggered by other sensory inputs'; that is, the up-close sights and sounds of the act of towel-folding. Michael Connor, 'Notes on ASMR, Massumi and the Joy of Digital Painting,' *Rhizome* (blog), May 8, 2013, http://rhizome.org/editorial/2013/may/08/notes-asmr-massumi-and-joy-digital-painting/
13. Renata Salecl, *Umbr(a) 1* (Buffalo, NY: The Center for the Study of Psychoanalysis & Culture, 1997), p. 106.
14. Lee Edelman, 'Stop Thinking about Tomorrow: Queerness, Ideology, and Anticipatory Democracy,' Lecture, Higgins School of Humanities Dialogue Symposium (Worcester, MA: Clark University), March 3, 2016.
15. Freud (2003), p. 141.
16. Ibid., p. 135.
17. 'Tingleheads' claim videos help ease stress,' *Today.com*, last modified October 15, 2014, http://www.today.com/health/tingleheads-claim-videos-help-ease-stress-2D80174447
18. '~•••~Relaxing Physical Therapist Visit~•••~,' *YouTube.com*, last modified January 6, 2013, https://www.youtube.com/watch?v=Hso5_Glnyx8&t=396s

19. 'patter, n.2,' *Oxford English Dictionary Online*, accessed February 15, 2017, http://goddard40.clarku.edu:2547/view/Entry/138972?rskey=F0NS1M&result=2#eid
20. 'patter, n.1,' *Oxford English Dictionary Online*, accessed February 15, 2017, http://goddard40.clarku.edu:2547/view/Entry/138971?result=1&rskey=F0NS1M&
21. 'patter, v.1,' *Oxford English Dictionary Online*, accessed February 15, 2017, http://goddard40.clarku.edu:2547/view/Entry/138973?
22. An interesting variation on classic ASMR roleplay patter is found in a video by YouTuber AccidentallyGraceful. Rather than improvising her dialogue, the speaker seems to have written out directions for making a cup of coffee using a French press, and then recites back the absurdly simplistic scripted directions in a calm, customary, perfectly enunciated monotone. Here again, the sense of rehearsal overrides that of real, caring interactivity. In similar videos by other YouTubers, mispronunciations and exaggerated foreign dialects only exacerbate this effect.
23. Historically, unintentional ASMR videos appeared first, and were collected in user lists before anyone thought to develop intentional roleplays. In 2017, however, roleplays clearly predominate.
24. 'Cranial Nerve Test with Pat LaFontaine & Dr. James Kelly,' *YouTube.com*, last modified April 28, 2011, https://www.youtube.com/watch?v=xrKbOF3vHo8
25. Cranial nerve exam videos are among the most popular forms of intentional ASMR roleplay, but various unintentional versions—including cranial nerve exam compilations—have long circulated in ASMR lists, on message boards, and so on.
26. 'About Us,' *Brainline.org*, accessed February 15, 2016, http://www.brainline.org/function_pages/about.html
27. Rob Gallagher, 'Eliciting Euphoria Online: The Aesthetics of "ASMR" Video Culture,' *Film Criticism* 40(4), 2016; accessed 15 Feb 2017, http://dx.doi.org/10.3998/fc.13761232.0040.202
28. '[Discussion] Misconceptions about ASMR Caused by High Participation of People Not Actually Experiencing It,' *Reddit.com*, accessed 15 Feb 2017, http://www.reddit.com/r/asmr/comments/4kkh1e/discussion_misconceptions_about_asmr_caused_by/
29. Steven Novella, 'ASMR,' *SkepticBlog* (blog), The Skeptics Society, March 12, 2012, http://www.skepticblog.org/2012/03/12/asmr/

30. Slavoj Žižek, *The Ticklish Subject: The Absent Centre of Political Ontology* (New York: Verso, 1999), p. 297.
31. Jacques Lacan, *Anxiety: The Seminar of Jacques Lacan, Book X*, ed. Jacques-Alain Miller, trans. A. R. Price (Cambridge, UK: Polity Press, 2014), p. 53.
32. Jacques-Alain Miller, 'Commentary on Lacan's Text,' in *Reading Seminars I and II*, eds. Richard Feldstein, Bruce Fink, and Maire Jaanus (Albany: SUNY Press, 2006), p. 423.
33. Gallagher (2016), np.

Bibliography

Connor, Michael. 2013. Notes on ASMR, Massumi and the Joy of Digital Painting. *Rhizome (blog)*, May 8. http://rhizome.org/editorial/2013/may/08/notes-asmr-massumi-and-joy-digital-painting/

Dolar, Mladen. 2006. *A Voice and Nothing More*. Cambridge: MIT Press.

Edelman, Lee. 2016. *Stop Thinking About Tomorrow: Queerness, Ideology, and Anticipatory Democracy*. Lecture, Higgins School of Humanities Dialogue Symposium. Clark University, Worcester, March 3.

Freud, Sigmund. 2003. *The Uncanny*. Trans. David McLintock. New York: Penguin Books.

Gallagher, Rob. 2016. Eliciting Euphoria Online: The Aesthetics of 'ASMR' Video Culture. *Film Criticism* 40(4): 1–15, http://dx.doi.org/10.3998/fc.13761232.0040.202. Accessed 15 Feb 2017.

Harari, Roberto. 2001. *Lacan's Seminar on Anxiety: An Introduction*. Trans. Jane C. Lamb-Ruiz. New York: Other Press.

Lacan, Jacques. 2014. *Anxiety: The Seminar of Jacques Lacan, Book X*, ed. Jacques-Alain Miller. Trans. A. R. Price. Cambridge: Polity Press.

Maslen, Hannah, and Rebecca Roache. 2015. ASMR and Absurdity. *Practical Ethics* (blog). University of Oxford, July 29, http://blog.practicalethics.ox.ac.uk/2015/07/asmr-and-absurdity/

Miller, Jacques-Alain. 2006. Commentary on Lacan's Text. In *Reading Seminars I and II*, ed. Richard Feldstein, Bruce Fink, and Maire Jaanus. Albany: SUNY Press.

Novella, Steven. 2012. ASMR. *SkepticBlog* (blog). The Skeptics Society, March 12. http://www.skepticblog.org/2012/03/12/asmr/

Salecl, Renata. 1997. *Umbr(a) 1*. Buffalo: The Center for the Study of Psychoanalysis & Culture.
Žižek, Slavoj. 1999. *The Ticklish Subject: The Absent Centre of Political Ontology*. New York: Verso.

For the Love of Nonhumanity: Anxiety, the Phallus, Transference, and Algorithmic Criticism

Jonathan Michael Dickstein

Humans and Nonhumans, Humanities and Nonhumanities

Interest in the nonhuman today has proliferated amid, and as an extension of, concerns about marginalized groups and voices. From the assumption that we should change our political situation, our immediate community, or even our psychological disposition to account better for otherness as a thing and an experience, research has inferred that this concept is radical and thus ought to be interrogated.[1] The humanistic response to the twenty-first century's mass corporatization of the academy represents a salient complement to these interrogations.[2] Noteworthy about the connection between the microanalysis of human–nonhuman relations and the macroanalysis of humanities–sciences relations, however, is that for the most part the latter tends to stress the difference involved while the prior tends to obscure it.[3] Given this misrelation between the microanalysis of the discipline's object (the human) vis-à-vis its Other

J.M. Dickstein (✉)
Independent Scholar, Worcester, MA, USA

G. Basu Thakur, J.M. Dickstein (eds.), *Lacan and the Nonhuman*,
The Palgrave Lacan Series, DOI 10.1007/978-3-319-63817-1_13

(the nonhuman) and the macroanalysis of the discipline (humanities) vis-à-vis its Other (the nonhumanities qua sciences), the question that emerges is: What exactly is the attribute that realizes the substantive distinction at stake?

Immediately, we must rule out that this attribute has anything to do with the object of the study itself because there exist obvious examples of nonhumanities that deal with the human, such as biology and (if we accept its position in the nonhumanities) psychology. Ruling out the object of the study, we find that the attribute should concern the study's approach or method. Debates pertaining to the scopes and aims of the digital humanities (i.e., as a living subset of the humanities) make this point thematic. Such debates reveal that the assumed impasse for the digital humanities is the excess made manifest by some irreducible human element—often referred to as 'cultural critique'—that any purely algorithmic qua nonhuman approach must fail to grasp.[4]

Nonetheless, Stephen Ramsay in his 2011 book, *Reading Machines*, tries to account for this seemingly ungraspable element by appealing to what he calls the 'essential' procedure of 'critical reading'—a procedure he develops according to a synthesis of Rob Pope's theory of 'textual intervention' (from his like-titled 1994 book) and the notion of 'deformance' of Lisa Samuels and Jerome McGann.[5] By demonstrating that this procedure is encodable, he attempts to found what he calls 'algorithmic criticism,' a culturally relevant form of computational literary analysis.

To make more precise the import and practice of this method, the present chapter aims to specify its stakes by reference to two related psychoanalytic notions: (1) anxiety, understood not as a confrontation that lacks an object but rather as a confrontation with a lacking object; and (2) transference, grasped epistemologically according to how one repeats resistance in a situation (whether clinical or not) to knowledge of one's desires. To demonstrate what is crucial to these stakes, this chapter reviews Lydia Liu's (re)interpretation of the cybernetic apparatus undergirding Jacques Lacan's initial (re)interpretation of Edgar Allan Poe's original (fantasmatic) account of Auguste Dupin's (re)interpretation of the logic surrounding the purloined letter in the 1844 'The Purloined Letter.' Conclusions are made regarding how what is called 'arithmocentrism' comes to confront one with the phallus, a confrontation suggesting a way by which computers might model the analytic experience.

What Algorithms Leave and/or Find Lacking

According to Ramsay, algorithmic criticism could proceed in steps akin to those students tend to appeal to when responding to the most common interpretative questions. He gives the example (by way of Pope) of questions instructors might ask when discussing Robert Browning's 1842 poem, 'My Last Duchess': '(1) how far personally are you prepared to adopt the Duke's position (his "voice" and self-image)?; (2) what other position(s) [do] you feel yourself drawn to adopt (even though they may have no "voices" or self-images directly available).'[6] As Ramsay explains:

> [S]tudents are led [like computers] to compose lists of the perspectives of voiceless and/or absent characters—ranging from the count's servant, the count and the count's daughter to the people who built the wall of the duke's chambers and those who tend the orchards beyond it—ultimately aiming to rewrite...the poem from a new center.'[7]

The conclusion Ramsay draws is that such a response amounts to a 'deformance' and may undergird an algorithmic criticism insofar as it represents 'nothing more than the basic textual maneuvers by which form gives way to form—the "de" functioning not as a privative, but as [a] relatively straightforward signifier of change.'[8]

Nevertheless, Ramsay's attempt here to prop up his own theory of algorithmic criticism by way of the broader notion of textual intervention qua deformance fails, not insofar as it is wrong, but rather insofar as it is much too universal. How, for example, does 'deformance' as being tantamount to 'maneuvers by which form gives way to form' differ from the scientific method—that is, making observations, formulating hypotheses about these observations, developing experiments for testing hypotheses about these observations, and drawing conclusions about the experiments for testing hypotheses about these observations? In addition, if deformance and the scientific method are the same, why develop a new word to name the latter (of course, other than for the mere sake of rhetorical embellishment)? The difficulty one faces in providing clear answers for these questions indicates that, although it might seem compelling, Ramsay's positioning of deformance as the modus operandi of textual criticism (also then the basis of algorithmic criticism) proves to lack any tangible theoretical ground to be beneficial.

Relief though comes when one considers a chief implication of Ramsay's work, which he himself indicates in passing during its course. As he writes, 'one wonders, given the nature of deformative activity, whether any critical act could ever be considered "incontestable," or if, given the rubric of objectivity, the movement from text to interpretation could ever be free of anxiety.'[9] In this context, a significant example of deformative activity, which Ramsay also discusses, is that of Chinua Achebe's 1977 article, 'An Image of Africa: Racism in Conrad's "Heart of Darkness,"' in which Achebe, to borrow the term of Ramsay and McGann/Samuels, deforms the novella by referring to the text as well as to Conrad's other writings and letters. This deformance is done in order to reveal the way this tale silences African characters, situating them not as people exploited by the Belgian Ivory-Trading Company but rather as meager background for Kurtz's decent into madness.[10] What distinguishes this deformance from a deformance of, for example, Browning's 'My Last Duchess,' which pertains to the way different characters experience the taste of the orchard's cherries, is not simply (as Ramsay indicates) the question of contestability, but more importantly the fact that it might (and did) produce a great deal of anxiety.[11]

Psychoanalysis provides a valuable model for grasping what such an experience entails. Furthermore, it develops a means for analyzing it by means of what it calls transference in and beyond the clinical setting—crucially (also uniquely, given the ordinary understanding of the latter notion) in the context of digital humanistic practices—thus representing in this process the viability of Ramsay's algorithmic criticism. To begin, we may find many of psychoanalysis' chief points about the experience of anxiety already in one of Sigmund Freud's earliest articles, 'On Grounds for Detaching a Particular Syndrome from Neurasthenia under the Description "Anxiety Neurosis"' (1895).[12] Fundamental in this piece is the claim that anxiety and anxiety neurosis are different insofar as the prior, as Freud notes, comprises 'all that is ordinarily spoken of as anxiousness—or a tendency to take a pessimistic view of things,' whereas the latter 'goes beyond a plausible anxiousness of this kind, and it is frequently recognized by the patient himself as a kind of compulsion.'[13] Freud clarifies this distinction in 'Inhibitions, Symptoms and Anxiety': 'Real danger is a danger that is known, and realistic anxiety is anxiety about a known danger of this sort. Neurotic anxiety is anxiety about an unknown danger. Neurotic danger is thus a danger that has still to be discovered.'[14]

Of additional importance when defining the unique characteristics of neurotic anxiety is its connection to sexuality. As Freud explicitly states in his 'A Reply to Criticisms of My Paper on Anxiety Neurosis' (1895), 'sexual factors play a predominant part and one which has been given far too little weight.'[15] Given the scope of the present chapter, however, a comprehensive discussion of these factors is not possible. Suffice it to say that in his early article he distinguishes between the genders in order to describe certain experiences that generate anxiety, experiences such as unmanageable abstinence or potency. Furthermore, in 'Inhibitions, Symptoms and Anxiety,' he goes into much more detail about the relationship between anxiety and libido, drawing a further distinction between 'instinctual (id-) anxiety' and 'ego-anxiety.'[16]

More meaningful in the present context is Freud's discussion of anxiety's singular relation to objects. As Freud declares in 'Inhibitions, Symptoms and Anxiety': 'Anxiety has an unmistakable relation to expectation; it is anxiety about something. It has a quality of indefiniteness and lack of object. In precise speech we use the word "fear" rather than "anxiety" if it has found an object.'[17] On the one hand, then, there is fear, which seems to have an object; it 'has found' it. On the other, there is anxiety, which seems to have none.

Jacques Lacan's intervention into the topic of anxiety hinges on this point. Although most scholars invoke the way Lacan, in this discussion and elsewhere, brings semiology to bear on Freudian psychoanalytic concepts, Lacan's much more far-reaching and consequential contributions to psychoanalytic teaching are his intricate epistemological considerations, those concerning anxiety's relation to objects being representative. As he explains in his seminar on anxiety (1962–1963), this experience does not lack an object; it is not a function without end. Rather, anxiety is that function, the object of which is missing. As he puts it, '*it is not without an object.*'[18] Precisely given English grammar, anxiety's object is a missing object—an object, to paraphrase Freud, that has not been found. Freud's original German text seems to complement this point given that in it he does not say 'anxiety has a quality of…lack of object' but rather of '*objektlosigkeit*' or objectlessness.[19]

There is a parallelism between this abstract noun and the other quality Freud attributes to anxiety—'*unbestimmtheit*' (i.e., indefiniteness or indeterminacy).[20] The alliterative alliance between this latter term and the German word for the unconscious, '*unbewusst*,' is unmistakable and ought to be stressed. A sort of semantic commutative affiliation then holds between *objeklosigkeit* and *unbewusst*. The significant difference is that the prior is explicitly an abstraction as is indicated by its suffix, '*keit*.' At stake, then, is a misrelation between the abstract and the concrete (i.e., concepts and objects).

In his 1964 seminar on the four fundamental concepts of psychoanalysis, Lacan provides a noteworthy frame for an understanding of this misrelation with the claim that 'there springs up a misunderstood form of the *un*, the *Un* of the *Unbewusste* [the unconscious]. Let us say that the limit of the *Unbewusste* is the *Unbegreff* [literally, un-concept]—not the non-concept, but the concept of lack.'[21] Being without an object does not entail that, as Lacan adds in his seminar on anxiety, 'one knows which object is involved.'[22] Negation and lack are distinct. For example, Lacan notes, '[w]hen I say, *He's not without resources, He's not without cunning*, it means, at least for me, that his resources are obscure, his cunning isn't run of the mill.'[23]

Lacan further suggests his appreciation for the stake of this distinction between negation and lack when he provides a linguistic interpretation of the function of the notion '*not without having*' according to the Latin triple negation '*non haud sine.*' He claims that '*haud*' operates as an apposition to '*sine*,' perhaps to intensify the indefiniteness of the negation presupposed by the latter term, yet also to connect it through the clear and precise verbal negation made manifest by the '*non*' to the existential and possessive lacks as in a phrase like '*est non haud sine habens* is.'[24]

Lacan demonstrates his awareness of the way the distinction between negation and lack pertains to the concept–object misrelation and thus bears on his understanding of anxiety when he concludes his disquisition with an outline of the sociological role the phallus plays. This is a role emphatically made abstract given his marking it with the capital Greek letter phi, Φ, which ironically, yet significantly, invokes Freud's own early deployment of this same letter to refer to the speculative subsystem of neurons that receives stimuli from the outside world (phi for physical or *physische* in German).[25]

The phallus for Lacan here has the purpose of being an object of 'social exchange' insofar as in what we ought to call the conceptual sexual relationship between man and woman it is only what can be guaranteed not to be lacking physically (i.e., castrated) from the man if it is possessed psychologically by the woman. Thus, anxiety as characterized by *objeklosigkeit*—now what we should redefine as the concept of a lacking object—is obviously experienced when this same man perceives the phallus 'fill[ing]…out' the woman's domain.[26]

The Rim That Could Be Transference

The psychoanalytic concept of 'transference' per Lacan's unique explanation of it relates explicitly to the discussion about anxiety and its connection to the phallus. Therefore, implicitly this same concept, given Lacan's explanation of it, pertains to the way anxiety concerns the humanistic method (i.e., deformance) undergirding the nonhumanistic process that is algorithmic criticism. Beginning with transference's more colloquial meaning, we might say that it refers to the event marking an analysand's or patient's development of feelings of love toward her or his analyst. In psychoanalytic literature, however, transference refers more broadly to events marking not only love but also hate and indifference—sometimes more significantly insofar as these events are produced by what are deemed rational or irrational motivations. Such distinctions find their expression in terms such as positive and negative transference—the prior indicating feelings of love and moreover, as Sigmund Freud suggests, sympathy, while the latter feelings of hate or distrust. They additionally pertain to contrasts like those between normal (i.e., rational) and neurotic (i.e., irrational) transference, the latter often referred to as 'transference neurosis.'

One would not be exaggerating if one were to suggest that transference is the most important concept of analytic technique, yet at the same time the most contested. The concept's level of importance is easily discernible in one of the earliest of Freud's psychoanalytic writings (cowritten with his mentor and cathartic psychologist Josef Breuer), *Studies on Hysteria* (1893–1895), where he introduces it in the context of a discussion of 'the important part played by the figure of the physician in creating motives to defeat the psychical force of resistance' here he was suggesting that transference amounts to a kind of displacement or projection 'to the figure of the physician the distressing ideas which arise in the content of analysis.' Such displacement or projection—that is, the unnoticed manifestation in the supposed final sessions of Breuer's treatment of Anno O—seemed (in Freud's view) to confirm the failure of this treatment.[27]

Freud continued to explore, expand on, formalize, and complicate the notion of transference throughout his writings, from other major early texts (i.e., his 1899 *The Interpretation of Dreams*) and his 1905 case study on *Dora*; to his formative essays, 'The Dynamics of Transference' (1912) and 'Observations on Transference-Love' (1915); to his later works dealing with the structural model of the unconscious (i.e., Id, Ego, and Superego), *Group Psychology and the Analysis of the Ego* (1921) and *The Question of Lay Analysis* (1926); and in his final years in 'Analysis Terminable and Interminable' (1937). In doing so, Freud situated the to-this-day contestable nature of the concept.

The major themes of this contestation, in the early though still foundational psychoanalytic literature, had to do with about six overarching topics: (1) whether transference is a unique process (i.e., *the* transference) or a polymorphic one (transferences); (2) whether and to what extent the subdivisions of it/them into rational/irrational (normal and neurotic transference), positive–negative, and real–imaginary make sense; (3) whether and to what extent it pertains to psychological archetypes; (4) whether it emerges only in the analytic situation and is in part produced/

suggested/encouraged by the analyst; (5) whether and in what sense its treatment has to do in the last instance with the patient's object(s) or ego; and, finally, (6) whether and in what sense its treatment concerns its opposite (i.e., countertransference).[28]

As with the topic of anxiety, Jacques Lacan interceded into such contestations about transference by stressing the epistemological frame for them given what he often described as the semiological features of the psyche and thereby of the unconscious, situating then, as he might have said, the dynamic registrations of transferential phenomena between the Symbolic and the Imaginary. His doing so entails that, as he explains in his 1960–1961 seminar on transference, attempts to grasp this phenomena according to the intersubjective relationship between patient/analysand and analyst always beg the question of the existence of the subject in connection with the thing of her or his desires or as actant at the helm of her or his (ideal) ego.[29]

What for Lacan is instead at stake in transference beyond or in place of these two poles of the intersubjective relation is the site of knowledge, grasped in his texts as a domain of Signifiers and nominated as the field of the capital Other. As he declares explicitly in Seminar XI on the four fundamental concepts of analysis (one of these concepts notably being transference), '[it is] unthinkable unless one sets out from the subject who is supposed to know.' The implication of this is that, as he claims earlier in the same seminar:

"Everything emerges from the structure of the signifier…[which] is based on what I first called the function of the cut and which is now articulated, in the development of my discourse [specifically in this context by reference to the Klein bottle named not after Melanie but the late nineteenth-century German mathematician Felix] as the topological function of the rim".[30] Notably, this rim divides domains just as the signifier splits the subject of knowledge such that the domains/knowledge present themselves as being no longer orientable according to a normative inside and outside of ordinary three-dimensional geometric settings.

The related, and in a sense equally important, effect of this refocusing of the intersubjective relation in terms of the subject's always already decentered epistemic correspondence with the capital Other is that the (still today) common positive psychological bifurcation of the realm of affects from the realm of intelligence does not hold. As Lacan points out in Seminar I on Freud's papers on technique, with explicit regard for the notion of transference: '[S]tarting off from the emotions, from the affective, from abreaction, and from other terms designating a certain number of the partitioned phenomena which indeed come about during analysis one nonetheless ends up…with something essentially intellectual,' demonstrating thereby the 'entirely superficial' qualities of distinctions between such beginnings and ends and the fact that such terms ought to be 'completely expunged from our papers.'[31] More fundamental for Lacan than this affective–intellectual divide is the experience of anxiety—the experience, as we determined earlier, '*not without an object*'—and, as in his 1959–1960 seminar on ethics, Lacan famously and paradoxically claims a direct connection to his complication of the affective–intellectual divide, the only '[affect] which does not deceive.'[32]

Most significant, though, is that in Lacan's view anxiety vis-à-vis transference presents itself not merely through 'the function of haste' or of a 'run[ning] headlong toward…resemblance in another,' but also in a conjunction with the field of desire as being the Other's desire.[33] He explains that we might construe anxiety as a 'danger signal,' warning the subject 'to get the hell out of there.'[34] Why? Because the object in question—the object of desire—makes manifest a threat. By manifesting a threat, however, this same object must be repressed (*zu Verdrangen*), revealing anxiety as more fundamentally a relationship between the subject and the place where this object once was—the place as the surrogate object of desire, an indeterminate (*unbestimmte*) object. At this level, anxiety amounts to 'the final or radical mode in which the subject continues to sustain his relationship to desire, even if it is an unbearable mode' according to the function of expectation (*Erwartung*)—a function the presentation of which, specifically during the manifestation of transference, the analyst comes to exemplify.[35]

Coming to exemplify the function of expectation, occupying the place where the object of desire once was, the analyst, faced with the analysand's anxiety in transference, acts in a way explicitly analogical to the way humanists do when interpreting a text. Nonetheless, we must not ourselves run headlong toward such resemblance. As Lacan declares in his seminar on anxiety, '[t]here doesn't have to be analysis for there to be transference…but transference without analysis is acting-out'—the latter in some sense, per Freud, being synonymous with repeating as distinct from remembering.[36] Lacan's point then appears to be that transference outside the clinical setting is merely a repetitious act, a nonspecific kind of compulsion. This point may seem accurate if we consider Norman Holland's attempt to bring this psychoanalytic concept to bear on literary critique; he writes: 'You may respond, as I do, to the driver behind you as a heavy father, and this is transference, nor am I out of it. And so with reading a poem. I may read it the way my mentors taught me, but I govern those processes just as I govern [my car].'[37]

Nevertheless, we ought to wonder with Lacan about the seeming distinction between a subject in a clinical setting and one outside it. For is not this difference undermined by Lacan's own explanation of the semiological structure underlying the human psyche? Insofar as Lacan is being consistent, we must understand his notion of transference without analysis as less an actual state of affairs than one localizable in his own system.[38] Transference with analysis, with an analyst, does not entail that there is another person, that there is an intersubjective relation, but rather that one discovers oneself, constructs oneself, out of joint and then comes to engage with this experience.

From Phallogocentrism to Arithmocentrism

Lacan's epistemological account of anxiety and transference with analysis, as opposed to transference without it, can therefore be applied to Samuels's and McGann's notion of 'deformance' and further thereby to Ramsay's conception of algorithmic criticism, to determine with more clarity the distinction between humanistic inquiry and its other side. Representative of this application is Lacan's interpretation of Edgar Allen Poe's 'The Purloined Letter,' which is notable in the current context for its own invocation of a nonhuman topic (i.e., cybernetics) in what ought to be called an anticipatory algorithmic framework.

The fact that Lacan's method has this latter quality should not be surprising because various other kinds of scholarly digital humanistic approaches (e.g., Franco Moretti's famous notion of distant reading and Jan Christoph Meister's formative account of computational narratology), whether explicitly or implicitly, owe their stakes to major ideological trends behind poststructuralism—that is, respectively, according to those two mentioned, Marxism and the Frankfurt School, as well as an intricate understanding of German Idealists (e.g., Johann Gottlieb Fichte and Georg Wilhelf Friedrich Hegel).[39] Lacan's interpretation of Poe's story similarly brings a unique appreciation for psychoanalytic concepts and techniques (also more or less indebted to Marxism and Hegelianism) to bear on proto-algorithmic hypotheses (i.e., early game theory).

The story by Poe of interest to Lacan builds on the detective style set up by Poe's preceding tales, 'The Murders of Rue Morgue' (1841) and 'The Mystery of Mary Rogêt' (1843), although it situates this style in a novel almost entirely dialogic narrative. As in its predecessors, nonetheless, the archetypical detective, the character Auguste Dupin, is central; his chief characteristic being that, as is explained in the earliest tale, he had 'a peculiar analytic ability' representing to the narrator a 'Bi-Part Soul' of 'the creative and the resolvent.'[40] Unlike in its predecessors, however, the mystery Dupin is charged to solve in the tale is no longer sensational, no longer therefore following the trend of Poe's noteworthy horror stories (i.e., the 1843 'The Black Cat' and 'Tell-Tale Heart'), but rather that of his more experimental pieces (i.e., the 1840 'The Man of the Crowd').[41] Specifically, the mystery Dupin is called on to tackle in 'The Purloined Letter' involves not murder but manners—the location of a handwritten message received by the Queen of France from an unnamed individual that contains material worthy of blackmail and that has been stolen by a Minister of the court.

Of chief importance to Lacan about this tale is less the totality of the narrative than one of its elements that has the diegetic, and also extradiegetic, characteristic of being this tale's key. On the one hand, this element represents a major basis for the method by which Dupin solves the mystery in question; on the other, it serves as a basis for the method by which Lacan interprets the tale and its implications. This element comes in the form of an anecdote enunciated by the perspicacious detective, an anecdote involving a childhood game designated the game 'of even and odd.'[42] As this detective explains, the 'game is simple, and is played with marbles. One player holds in his hand a number of these; and demands of another whether that number is even or odd. If the guess is right, the guesser wins one; if wrong, he loses one.'[43] A boy at school proved an expert at this game because of a 'principle of guessing'—a principle based on a '*thorough* identification' of his opponent's intellect by 'fashion[ing] the expression' of his own face 'in accordance with the expression' of this opponent's and 'wait[ing] to see what thoughts or sentiments arise in [his] mind or heart, as if to match or correspond with the expression.'[44]

What for Lacan is essential to this anecdote is the relation of knowledge that it exemplifies and that manifests itself again at the level of the tale's narrative. His interpretation of this relation may be reduced to a lengthy passage where he describes the two fundamental scenes of Poe's story, the first entitled, significantly, 'the primal scene' and the second 'its repetition' in the sense crucial to the psychoanalytic notion of repetition automatism or acting out.[45] Lacan concludes this passage by outlining the three fundamental components of the scenes that repeat: (1) 'a glance that sees nothing: the King and the police'; (2) 'a glance which sees that the first sees nothing and deludes itself as to the secrecy of what it hides: the Queen, then the Minister'; and (3) '[a glance that sees] the first two glances leave what should be hidden exposed to whomever would seize it: the Minister, and finally Dupin.'[46]

After he outlines these components, Lacan briefly considers their implications in terms of what he calls '*la politique de l'autruiche*' (the politics of the ostrich, significantly with a homological relation to a *politique de l'autre* or politics of the Other).[47] These implications amount to the fact that a middle or second party believes itself invisible or imperceptible because the front, or first, has its head stuck in the ground, although in this belief lets a final or third party 'pluck its rear.'[48]

Critics, such as Jacques Derrida and Barbara Johnson, despite their intricacies and import, focus almost exclusively on the structure of this interpretation and the value or problems with Lacan's interpretation of it. On a surface level, in 'The Purveyor of Truth' (1975), Derrida locates in its supposed triadic logic the essence of what he terms 'phallogocentrism,' the starting point for which is 'a determinate situation...in which the phallus is the mother's desire insasmuch as she does not have it.'[49] As Johnson explains, 'the problem with psychoanalytical triangularity, in Derrida's eyes, is not that it contains the wrong number of terms, but that it presupposes the possibility of a successful dialectical mediation and harmonious normalization or Aufhebung [more often, sublation] of desire.'[50] Still, Johnson notes how Derrida's own account of Lacan's interpretation is itself oversimplified and often repetitious of claims already manifest in the latter. Thus, she argues that 'the more one works with Derrida's analysis, the more convinced one becomes that…it does not quite apply to what Lacan's text is actually saying. What Derrida is in fact arguing against is therefore not Lacan's text but Lacan's power.'[51]

Focusing on the structure inherent to the logic of Lacan's text though seems to miss the real consequence of his concerns—namely, that the heart of the logic of Poe's tale has an explicit affinity with cybernetics and, more broadly, automation. As Lacan explains just after reviewing the so-called game of odd and even in his 1954–1955 seminar on the ego, initially one suspects the import of the game amounts to 'a matter of simple psychological penetration, a kind of egomiming.'[52] Nevertheless, such a suspicion 'already presupposes the dimension of intersubjectivity' because the one player must 'know that he is faced with another subject, in principle homogeneous with him.'[53] Therefore, this suspicion is 'totally inadequate'; another rigorously 'logical' path is necessary.[54]

Lacan discerns this path in the fact that it manifests itself as soon as one's opponent 'is the machine.'[55] As he explains:

> It is clear that you don't have to ask yourself whether the machine is stupid or intelligent, whether it will play in accordance with its first or its second go. Inversely, the machine has no means of placing itself in a reflexive position in relation to its human partner. …/ The physiognomy of the machine, however prepossessing it may be, can be of no help whatsoever. …No means of getting out of it by way of identification. One is thus from the start forced to take the path of language [*langage*], of the possible combinatory of the machine.[56]

That per Lacan's interpretation here Poe's tale warrants a kind of combinatory, cybernetic, or, to invoke Ramsay, algorithmic critique, should not be surprising given Poe's own critical studies, such as 'The Philosophy of Composition' (1846), 'The Rationale of Verse' (1848), and 'The Poetic Principle' (1850). The 1846 study, for example, provides a rigorous formal analysis of Poe's own poem, 'The Raven' (1845), in terms of nearly all its structural qualities—from its rhythm and rhyme to the motivation underlying the selection of the 'or' sound of the famous repeated term 'nevermore.'[57] Lacan's interpretation of the cybernetic undercurrents of Poe's 'The Purloined Letter' seems to bring a similar goal into a more modern sphere.[58]

Thus, as Lydia Liu explains in her 2010 article, 'The Cybernetic Unconscious: Rethinking Lacan, Poe, and French Theory':

> [A] common mistake [has been]...to fetishize Lacan's textual excursions in the 'Seminar on "The Purloined Letter"' as a virtuoso performance in psychoanalytic criticism and turn that criticism into all kinds of navel-gazing exercises. Such exercises have had the unfortunate consequence of thwarting the political decision or intuition that had gone into Lacan's adoption of Poe's text and thereby deflecting his important discoveries concerning the Freudian unconscious.[59]

Undoubtedly, Liu has in mind such critics of Lacan's interpretation of this story (e.g., Derrida's and Johnson's), who frame their argument with questions, such as 'what occurs in the psychoanalytical deciphering of a text when the deciphered (text), already explains itself.' —as Derrida writes, 'evidences itself'—in this deciphering.[60] Perhaps though it is this auto-explaining, this auto-evidencing, that the analyst in question (Lacan) ought to have found significant, when in the context of transference, he must have come to exemplify the function of expectation and thereby to occupy the place of the lacking or, to follow the emergent themes, purloined object of desire. Therefore, the result might have been a realization of the experience of anxiety so readily reducible in our present state of affairs to the alternating Symbolic–Imaginary operations of the phallus.

Setting the stage for an appreciation of this point, Liu further assesses the cybernetic (i.e., nonhuman) undercurrent of Poe's story per Lacan's original interpretation of it, meticulously tracing the way that notably American cyberneticists have in a sense been '*hiding in plain sight*' to critics of Lacan's interpretation of Poe's tale.[61] That such an assessment amounts to a deformance—a reformation of the original text in question that has the potential to produce anxiety—is clear. Its own connection to algorithmic critique is equally obvious if we consider the details it reviews about cybernetics and moreover the way Lacan proceeds in his seminar to articulate the scansion of the machine's combinatory potential in the context of the odd–even game.

To expedite the conclusion of the current chapter, though, such intricacies are not able to be reviewed; rather only the lessons they imply are. In the first place, Liu poses a question clearly deformative (in our nuanced sense of the term) and essential to cybernetics and Lacan's interpretation of Poe's tale alike:

> Does the mind behave like a telephone exchange system or is it also a machine? ...[Various cyberneticists have] answered yes, for cybernetics was premised on the idea that communication networks and neural pathways corresponded to each other in more than analogical ways. Lacan came very close to answering 'yes' as he speculated further about the nature of language and of the unconscious by reference to the cybernetic machine.[62]

Liu here demonstrates her desire to challenge the possibility of an identification between human and machine, human and nonhuman, and situates Lacan at the border between the right and the wrong action. She reiterates this same appeal in her concluding remarks, deciding though that Lacan ultimately selects the right course: 'Will the theory of language and the theory of the unconscious be the same after the arrival of cybernetics? Lacan's answer is no, and he is right. The originality of his work lies precisely in its radical openness toward the temporality of "what appears in our world."'[63]

If Liu's point then is deformative of a text, however, it is deformative of Lacan's text. But then again, Lacan's text too is deformative, situating an experience of anxiety based on an interpretation of Poe's tale evidenced by the critical but also approving responses he received. Essential to Lacan's 'deformance' is the fact that it brings humans face to face with their supposed Other—the machine, the nonhuman. One need only glance further at Derrida's 1975 article to recognize that beyond the problematic of the phallogocentric dialectic is an androcentric one (i.e., a purely masculinist position that supersedes its physical bases).[64] In a similar way, Johnson finds disconcerting the possibility of what might be called a sterile exchange: '[I]f the complexities of these texts [Derrida's, Lacan's, Poe's] could be reduced to a mere combat between ostriches, a mere game of heads and tails played out in order to determine a "winner," they would have very little theoretical interest.'[65] Furthermore, Liu's concern about the potential that Lacan could have answered 'yes' to the question—is the mind a machine?—additionally demonstrates how the threat of the nonhuman is recognized yet tamed.

Crucial to stress is that the phallus in these scenarios, as the function of an indeterminate object signaling anxiety, fails to show itself in phallocentrism, phallogocentrism, androcentrism, and also opposing positions like gynocentrism, androgynocentrism, gynoandrocentrism, extra-gynoandrocentrism, and so on. Generally, the phallus as what might be called the unsaturated place for the indeterminate object of anxiety does not appear in any situation or discourse of its pure centering or pure decentering but instead only in a framework or model of its original displacement, what might be called arithmocentrism—where what Derrida refers to as the 'determinate *situation*' is exponentially multiplied, coming thereby to inspire various logics of desire each in different but related ways emerging out of joint.

(Sie)Er/Es Lässt Sich Nicht Lessen

The essence of humanistic interpretation may be understood in terms of deformance, and deformance may be qualified in terms of the anxiety it produces. Furthermore, algorithmic criticism may be grasped as what is able to act out deformance, and this love of nonhumanity acted out by alogirthmic criticism, acted out by digital humanities, may be analyzed as itself deformative vis-à-vis the discipline or set of disciplines it deems its home. Therefore, we humanists (digital or otherwise) must realize that we always operate (more or less with clarity) according to transference insofar as here the nonhuman presents itself there where we are in the form of the phallus, encoded by the uppercase symbol Φ, and exemplified by some sourceless, nonorientable expression, like the one framing Poe's aforementioned, though undiscussed, less-sensational, detective-like tale, 'The Man of the Crowd.' This expression reads: '[*(sie)*]*er[/es] lässt sich nicht lessen*'—(s)he/it permits itself not to be read.[66]

Notes

1. See, for example, Judith Butler, *Undoing Gender* (New York: Routledge, 2004), pp. 12, 30; Jane Bennett, *Vibrant Matter: A Political Ecology of Things* (Durham, NC: Duke University Press, 2010)., p. xvi.
2. Consider Stanley Fish, 'The Crisis of the Humanities Official Arrives' (2010), NYTimes.com, https://opinionator.blogs.nytimes.com/2010/10/11/the-crisis-of-the-humanities-officially-arrives/?_r=0 (accessed 1 Nov 2016); and Steven Pearlstein, 'Meet the Parents Who Won't Let Their Children Study Literature' (2016), WashingtonPost.com, https://www.washingtonpost.com/posteverything/wp/2016/09/02/meet-the-parents-who-wont-let-their-children-study-literature/?utm_term=.68d0d86b3c3b (accessed 1 Nov 2016).
3. Fish, for example, claims that to remedy the so-called 'crisis' of the humanities professionals must 'explain and defend' without apology that humanities situate has a 'core enterprise' separate and distinct from the sciences and must continue to do so (Fish 2010). Pearlstein suggests in his conclusion similarly, though more pointedly, that one who 'spends four years contemplating the meaning of life…[at least] won't make the mistake of confusing the meaning of life with maximizing lifetime income' (Pearlstein 2016).
4. For a basic understanding of the stakes of these debates, see Stephen Ramsay, 'Who's In and Who's Out' (2011b) *StephenRamsay.us*, http://stephenramsay.us/text/2011/01/08/whos-in-and-whos-out/ (accessed 1 Nov 2016); and a transcription of Ramsay's piece from the formative 2011 Modern Language Association panel, 'History and Future of Digital Humanities,' chaired by Kathleen Fitzpatrick. See also Mark Sample's salient response, 'The Digital Humanities Is Not About Building, It's About Sharing' (2011), *SampleReality.com*, http://www.samplereality.com/2011/05/25/the-digital-humanities-is-not-about-building-its-about-sharing/ (accessed 1 Nov 2016). Similarly, see Fish, 'Mind Your P's and B's: The Digital Humanities and Interpretation' (2012), NYTimes.com, https://opinionator.blogs.nytimes.com/2012/01/23/mind-your-ps-and-bs-the-digital-humanities-and-interpretation/ (accessed 1 Nov 2016); and Ramsay's response 'Stanley and Me' (2012) StephenRamsay.us, http://stephenramsay.us/text/2012/11/08/stanley-and-me/ (accessed 1 Nov 2016). For a broader appreciation of the debates in question, see *Debates in Digital Humanities* (Minneapolis: University of Minnesota Press, 2012, 2016).

5. Ramsay, *Reading Machines* (Chicago: University of Illinois Press, 2011a), p. xi. See also Rob Pope, *Textual Intervention: Critical and Creative Strategies for Literary Studies* (New York: Routledge, 1994); and Lisa Samuels and Jerome McGann, 'Deformance and Interpretation,' *New Literary History* 20(1): 25–56, 1999.
6. Pope (1994), p. 15 qtd., in Ramsay (2011), p. 33.
7. Ramsay (2011a), p. 33.
8. Ibid., p. 56.
9. Ibid., p. 49.
10. Cf. Chinua Achebe, 'An Image of Africa: Racism in Conrad's "Heart of Darkness,"' *Heart of Darkness* (New York: W. W Norton, 2016), pp. 306–320.
11. Note that this point does not entail that an interpretation of Browning's poem does not yield anxiety. For an instructive example, consider W.T.J. Mitchell's account in 'Representation,' *Critical Terms for Literary Study* (Chicago: University of Chicago Press, 1990), pp. 11–22.
12. Freud would restate many of the points from this early article throughout the proceeding four or so decades of his career and life in more canonical texts, such as *The Interpretation of Dreams* (1899) (i.e., with the topic of anxiety-dreams), *Introductory Lectures on Psychoanalysis* (1916–1917), *Group Psychology and the Analysis of the Ego* (1921), and most notably 'Inhibitions, Symptoms and Anxiety' (1926).
13. Sigmund Freud, 'On Grounds for Detaching a Particular Syndrome from Neurasthenia under the Description "Anxiety Neurosis"' (1895), *The Complete Psychological Works of Sigmund Freud, Vol. III*, ed. James Strachey (London: Hogarth Press, 1962b), p 93.
14. Freud, 'Inhibitions, Symptoms and Anxiety' (1926), *The Complete Psychological Works of Sigmund Freud, Vol. XX*, ed. James Strachey (London: Hogarth Press, 1959a), p. 164.
15. Freud, 'A Reply to Criticisms of My Paper on Anxiety Neurosis' (1895), *The Complete Psychological Works of Sigmund Freud, Vol. III*, ed. James Strachey (London: Hogarth Press, 1962a), p 123.
16. Freud (1959a), p. 160. The complex and perhaps problematic distinction Freud makes between object and ego libido is also at issue here. This distinction further connects to the famously controversial contrast he draws between castration anxiety and penis envy. Regarding these topics, a reader skpetical of Freud's seemingly essentialistic biologism might compare Freud, *Three Essays on Sexuality* (1903), *The Complete Psychological Works of Sigmund Freud, Vol. VII*, ed. James Strachey

(London: Hogarth Press, 1953), pp. 125–243 and Freud, 'On Narcissism' (1914), *The Complete Psychological Works of Sigmund Freud, Vol. XIV,* ed. James Strachey (London Hogarth Press, 1957), pp. 67–102. Also, Jamieson Webster's chapter in the current volume, 'Toward a Less-Than-Human Psychoanalysis: Coitus Interruptus and the Object,' discusses similar themes in much more depth.
17. Ibid., pp. 163–164.
18. Jacques Lacan, *The Seminar of Jacques Lacan, Book X: Anxiety (1962–1963)*, trans. A. R. Price (Cambridge, UK: Polity, 2014), p. 89; italics in original.
19. Freud (1959a), p. 164; in Freud, *Gesammelte Werke, Band XIV* (London: Imago Publishing, 1991), p. 196.
20. Ibid.
21. Lacan, *The Seminar of Jacques Lacan, Book XI: The Four Fundamental Concepts of Psychoanalysis* (1964), trans. Alan Sheridan (New York: W. W. Norton, 1981), p. 26.
22. Lacan (2014), p. 89.
23. Ibid.
24. Ibid; italics in original.
25. Ibid.; cf. Freud, *Project for a Scientific Psychology (1950 [1895]), The Complete Psychological Works of Sigmund Freud, Vol. I*, ed. James Strachey (London: Hogarth Press, 1966), pp. 281–391. Perhaps notable is that Freud uses the lowercase phi.
26. Ibid.
27. Freud, *Studies on Hysteria (1893–1895), The Complete Psychological Works of Sigmund Freud, Vol. II*, ed. James Strachey (London: Hogarth Press, 1955), pp. 301–302.
28. Ida Macalpine, 'The Development of the Transference,' *The Psychoanalytic Quarterly*19): 501–539, 1950. This article elaborates on some of these discussions (following the order I developed) by reference to for (2) William Silverberg's *The Concept of Transference* (1948), Sandor Ferenczi's 'Introjection and Transference,' (1909), Otto Fenichel's *Problems of Psychoanalytic Technique* (1941), and Franz Alexander's and Thomas French's *Psychoanalytic Therapy* (1946); and for (5) Melanie Klein's 'Symposium on Child-Analysis' (1927) and Anna Freud's *The Ego and the Mechanisms of Defense* (1936). Per references from Lacan, *The Seminar of Jacques Lacan, Book VIII: Transference (1960–1961),* trans. Bruce Fink (Cambridge, UK: Polity, 2015) and per notoriety, I summoned for (2), Herman Nunberg's 'Transference and Reality' (1951) and Thomas

Szasz's 'The Concept of Transference' (1963); for (3) Carl Jung's *The Psychology of Transference* (1946), Lola Paulsen's 'Transference and Projection' (1956); for (5) Clara Thompson's 'Transference as a Therapeutic Treatment' (1945) and her 'The Role of the Analyst's Personality in Therapy' (1956); for (6) Roger Money-Kyrle's 'Normal Countertransference and Some of Its Deviations' (1956) and Cecil Patterson's 'Transference and Countertransference' (1959).

29. Lacan (2015), pp. 314–315.
30. Lacan (1981), pp. 253, 206.
31. Lacan, *The Seminar of Jacques Lacan, Book I: Freud's Papers on Technique (1953–1954)*, trans. John Forrester (New York: W. W. Norton, 1991a), pp. 281, 275.
32. Lacan (2014), p. 89; Lacan, *The Seminar of Jacques Lacan, Book VII: The Ethics of Psychoanalysis (1959–1960)*, trans. Dennis Porter (New York: W. W. Norton, 1997), p. 41.
33. Lacan (2015), p. 363.
34. Ibid.
35. Ibid., pp. 365, 362.
36. Lacan (1997), p. 125. Cf. also Freud, 'Remembering, Repeating and Working-Through' (1914), *The Complete Psychological Works of Sigmund Freud, Vol. XII*, ed. James Strachey (London: Hogarth Press, 1958c), p. 151.
37. Norman Holland, 'Why This Is Transference, Nor Am I Out of It,' *Psychoanalysis and Contemporary Thought* 5: 29, 1982.
38. Cf. Freud, 'The Question of Lay Analysis (1926),' *The Complete Psychological Works of Sigmund Freud, Vol. XX*, ed. James Strachey (London: Hogarth Press, 1959b), pp. 179–270. My point here may seem more radical than Freud's as there is no question of training at all (medical or otherwise). On this radicalism, cf. further Freud, 'Recommendations to Physicians Practising Psycho-Analysis' (1912), *The Complete Psychological Works of Sigmund Freud, Vol. XII*, ed. James Strachey (London: Hogarth Press, 1958b), pp. 109–120. Similarly, one might observe that the theme concerning who is and who is not an analyst (likewise, who is able to be one) was a theme considered by Lacan throughout his teachings. At one point, for example, Lacan observes that knowing everything about psychoanalysis does not make one an analyst, specifically because analysis itself is not a complete domain (i.e., how could anyone know everything about it and, as important, what sort of person would claim to do so?). Jacques-Alain Miller's position in and/or

out of the field during the time when he first entered it and also still today is (I think) paradigmatic in this context.

39. Cf. Franco Moretti, *Distant Reading* (Brooklyn: Verso, 2013); and Jan Christoph Meister, *Computing Action: A Narratological Approach*, trans. Alastair Matthews (New York: Walter de Gruyter, 2003).
40. Edgar Allan Poe, 'The Murders in the Rue Morgue' (1841), *Standard Edition of the Works of Edgar Allan Poe, Vol. I*, ed. John H. Ingram (London: A & C Black, 1899), p. 409.
41. Walter Benjamin has discussed the stylistic similarities between 'The Man of the Crowd' and Poe's detective fiction. Cf. Benjamin, *Charles Baudelaire: A Lyrical Poet in the Era of High Capitalism*, trans. Harry Zohn (London: Verso, 1997). Relatedly, Charles Baudelaire has considered this short tale 'a picture…written' in 'III. The Artist, Man of the World, Man of the Crowd, and Child,' *The Painter of Modern Life*, trans. Jonathan Mayne (London: Phaidon Press, 1995), p. 7. In extension, one perhaps wonders about the connections among Poe's detective fiction, his pseudo-detective fiction, and his satires. Considerations in this context might be given to Poe's earlier 'The Man That Was Used Up' (1938) and 'The Business Man' (1940), *Standard Edition of the Works of Edgar Allan Poe, Vol. II*, ed. John H. Ingram (London: A & C Black, 1899), pp. 549–569.
42. Poe, 'The Purloined Letter' (1844), *Standard Edition of the Works of Edgar Allan Poe, Vol. I*, ed. John H. Ingram (London: A & C Black, 1899), pp. 503–504.
43. Poe (1844), p. 504.
44. Ibid.
45. Lacan, 'Seminar on "The Purloined Letter"' (1956), trans. Jeffrey Mehlman, *Yale French Studies* 48: 41, 1972.
46. Lacan (1972), p. 44.
47. Ibid. Cf. Freud's notion of the 'ostrich policy' or 'der Taktik des Vogels' in 'The Interpretation of Dreams (Second Part) (1900–1901),' *The Complete Psychological Works of Sigmund Freud, Vol. V*, ed. James Strachey (London: Hogarth Press, 1958a), p. 600.
48. Lacan (1972), p. 44.
49. Jacques Derrida, 'The Purveyor of Truth,' trans. Willis Domingo, James Hulbert, Moshe Ron, and M.-R. L., *Yale French Studies* 52: 98–99, 1975. Cf. also Gilles Deleuze, *Anti-Oedipus*, trans. Robert Hurley (New York: Penguin Classics, 2009).

50. Barbara Johnson, 'The Frame of Reference: Poe, Lacan, Derrida,' *Yale French Studies* 55–56: 472, 1977.
51. Ibid., p. 477.
52. Lacan, *The Seminar of Jacques Lacan, Book II: The Ego in Freud's Theory and in the Technique of Psychoanalysis (1954–1955)*, trans. Sylvana Tomaselli (New York: W. W. Norton, 1991b), p. 180.
53. Ibid.
54. Lacan (1991a), p. 181.
55. Ibid.
56. Ibid.
57. Poe, 'The Philosophy of Composition' (1841), *Standard Edition of the Works of Edgar Allan Poe, Vol. III*, ed. John H. Ingram (London: A & C Black, 1899), p. 271.
58. Worth noting may be that Lacan does remain committed to the combinatory potential of the machine, a counting-up tactic that proceeds from a starting point (the plus and minus dichotomy). A conversation I had with a software designer demonstrated that one must also account for what one might call the counting-down possibility inherent in the fact that the machine can (be encoded to) cheat. Specifically, before one selects marbles from one's own pile, the machine could survey the total number there so that, after one selects one's marbles, the machine could subtract the number to know without doubt whether your sum is odd or even.
59. Lydia Liu, 'The Cybernetic Unconscious: Rethinking Lacan, Poe, and French Theory,' *Critical Inquiry* 36(2): 289, Winter 2010. Cf. also Liu, *The Freudian Robot: Digital Media and the Future of the Unconscious* (Chicago: University of Chicago Press, 2011).
60. Derrida (1975), p. 32.
61. Liu (2010), p. 318; italics in original.
62. Ibid., pp. 315–316.
63. Ibid., p. 320.
64. Derrida (1975), p. 98.
65. Johnson (1977), p. 468.
66. Poe, 'Man in the Crowd' (1840), *Standard Edition of the Works of Edgar Allan Poe, Vol. II*, ed. John H. Ingram (London: A & C Black, 1899), pp. 314, 323. The German phrase here and in the subtitle is modified to reflect the original English translation Poe gave: 'it does not permit itself to be read.'. Oddly, according to the tale, 'er' refers to a book (in German, *das Buch*). Perhaps Poe had in mind the author of the book (*der Autor des*

Buches)—of course, given the pronoun's functioning, a male author. To capture these (in)decisions, along with the modified German subtitle and quotation are added the 'he' signalling the correct translation of the original pronoun and also the parenthetical 's' as a token of what was already elided in the phrase by the (un)intentional 'r' that might be said to exemplify how a letter always arrives at its destination insofar as it rips into that place where it fails to stand.

Bibliography

Achebe, Chinua. 2016. An Image of Africa: Racism in Conrad's 'Heart of Darkness'. In *Heart of Darkness*, 306–320. New York: W. W Norton.

Alexander, Franz, and Thomas French. 1980. *Psychoanalytic Therapy (1946)*. Lincoln: Bison Book.

Baudelaire, Charles. 1995. *The Painter of Modern Life*. Trans. Jonathan Mayne. London: Phaidon Press.

Benjamin, Walter. 1997. *Charles Baudelaire: A Lyrical Poet in the Era of High Capitalism*. Trans. H. Zohn. London: Verso.

Bennett, Jane. 2010. *Vibrant Matter: A Political Ecology of Things*. Durham: Duke University Press.

Butler, Judith. 2004. *Undoing Gender*. New York: Routledge.

Deleuze, Gilles. 2009. *Anti-Oedipus*. Trans. R. Hurley. New York: Penguin Classics.

Derrida, Jacques. 1975. The Purveyor of Truth. Trans. Willis Domingo, James Hulbert, Moshe Ron, and M.-R. L. *Yale French Studies* 52: 31–113.

Fenichel, Otto. 1969. *Problems of Psychoanalytic Technique (1941)*. Trans. David Brunswick. New York: Psychoanalytic Quarterly Press.

Ferenczi, Sandor. 1916. Introjection and Transference. In *Contributions to Psychoanalysis*, pp. 30–79. Trans. E. Jones. Boston: Richard G. Badger.

Fish, Stanley. 2010. The Crisis of the Humanities Official Arrives. *NYTimes.com*. https://opinionator.blogs.nytimes.com/2010/10/11/the-crisis-of-the-humanities-officially-arrives/?_r=0. Accessed 1 Nov 2016.

———. 2012. Mind Your P's and B's: The Digital Humanities and Interpretation. *NYTimes.com*. https://opinionator.blogs.nytimes.com/2012/01/23/mind-your-ps-and-bs-the-digital-humanities-and-interpretation/. Accessed 1 Nov 2016.

Freud, Anna. 1992. *The Ego and the Mechanisms of Defense (1936)*. London: Karnac Books.

Freud, Sigmund. 1953. Three Essays on Sexuality (1903). In *The Complete Psychological Works of Sigmund Freud*, ed. James Strachey, vol. VII, 125–243. London: Hogarth Press.

———. 1955. Studies on Hysteria (1893–1895). In *The Complete Psychological Works of Sigmund Freud, Vol. II*, ed. James Strachey, pp. 301–302. London: Hogarth Press.

———. 1957. On Narcissism' (1914). In *The Complete Psychological Works of Sigmund Freud*, ed. James Strachey, vol. XIV, 67–102. London: Hogarth Press.

———. 1958a. The Interpretation of Dreams (Second Part) (1900–1901). In *The Complete Psychological Works of Sigmund Freud, Vol. V*, ed. James Strachey, pp. ix–627. London: Hogarth Press.

———. 1958b. Recommendations to Physicians Practising Psycho-Analysis (1912). In *The Complete Psychological Works of Sigmund Freud*, ed. James Strachey, vol. XII, 109–120. London: Hogarth Press.

———. 1958c. Remembering, Repeating and Working-Through (1914). In *The Complete Psychological Works of Sigmund Freud*, ed. James Strachey, vol. XII, 145–156. London: Hogarth Press.

———. 1959a. Inhibitions, Symptoms and Anxiety (1926). In *The Complete Psychological Works of Sigmund Freud, Vol. XX*, ed. James Strachey, 75–176. London: Hogarth Press.

———. 1959b. The Question of Lay Analysis (1926). In *The Complete Psychological Works of Sigmund Freud, Vol. XX*, ed. James Strachey, pp. 179–270. London: Hogarth Press.

———. 1962a. A Reply to Criticisms of My Paper on Anxiety Neurosis (1895). In *The Complete Psychological Works of Sigmund Freud, Vol. III*, ed. James Strachey, 119–139. London: Hogarth Press.

———. 1962b. On Grounds for Detaching a Particular Syndrome from Neurasthenia under the Description "Anxiety Neurosis" (1895). In *The Complete Psychological Works of Sigmund Freud, Vol. III*, ed. James Strachey, 85–115. London: Hogarth Press.

———. 1966. Project for a Scientific Psychology (1950 [1895]). *The Complete Psychological Works of Sigmund Freud, Vol. I*, ed. James Strachey, pp. 281–391. London: Hogarth Press.

Gold, Matthew K., ed. 2012. *Debates in Digital Humanities*. Minneapolis: University of Minnesota Press.

Gold, Matthew K., and Lauren F. Klein, eds. 2016. *Debates in Digital Humanities*. Minneapolis: University of Minnesota Press.

Holland, Norman. 1982. Why This Is Transference, Nor Am I Out of It. *Psychoanalysis and Contemporary Thought* 5: 27–34.

Johnson, Barbara. 1977. The Frame of Reference: Poe, Lacan, Derrida. *Yale French Studies* 55–56: 28–47.

Jung, Carl. 1983. *The Psychology of the Transference* (1954). Trans. R.F.C. Hull. New York: Routledge.

Klein, Melanie. 1975. Symposium on Child-Analysis (1927). In *Love, Guilt and Reparation and Other Works*, pp. 139–169. New York: The Free Press.

Lacan, Jacques. 1972. Seminar on 'The Purloined Letter' (1956). Trans. Jeffrey Mehlman. *Yale French Studies* 48: 41.

———. 1981. *The Seminar of Jacques Lacan, Book XI: The Four Fundamental Concepts of Psychoanalysis (1964)*. Trans. Alan Sheridan. New York: W. W. Norton.

———. 1991a. *The Seminar of Jacques Lacan, Book I: Freud's Papers on Technique (1953–1954)*. Trans. John Forrester. New York: W. W. Norton.

———. 1991b. *The Seminar of Jacques Lacan, Book II: The Ego in Freud's Theory and in the Technique of Psychoanalysis (1954–1955)*. Trans. Sylvana Tomaselli. New York: W. W. Norton.

———. 1997. *The Seminar of Jacques Lacan, Book VII: The Ethics of Psychoanalysis (1959–1960)*. Trans. Dennis Porter. New York: W. W. Norton.

———. 2014. *The Seminar of Jacques Lacan, Book X: Anxiety (1962–1963)*. Trans. A. R. Price. Cambridge: Polity.

———. 2015. *The Seminar of Jacques Lacan, Book VIII: Transference (1960–1961)*. Trans. Bruce Fink. Cambridge: Polity.

Liu, Lydia. 2010. The Cybernetic Unconscious: Rethinking Lacan, Poe, and French Theory. *Critical Inquiry* 36 (2): 288–320.

———. 2011. *The Freudian Robot: Digital Media and the Future of the Unconscious*. Chicago: University of Chicago Press.

Macalpine, Ida. 1950. The Development of the Transference. *The Psychoanalytic Quarterly* 19: 501–539.

Meister, Jan Christoph. 2003. *Computing Action: A Narratological Approach*. Trans. A. Matthews. New York: Walter de Gruyter.

Mitchell, W.T.J. 1990. Representation. In *Critical Terms for Literary Study*, 11–22. Chicago: University of Chicago Press.

Money-Kyrle, Roger E. 1956. Normal Counter-Transference and Some of Its Deviations. *The International Journal of Psychoanalysis* 37: 360–366.

Moretti, Franco. 2013. *Distant Reading*. Brooklyn: Verso.

Nunberg, Herman. 1951. Transference and Reality. *The International Journal of Psychoanalysis* 32: 1–9.

Patterson, Cecil. 1959. *Counseling and Psychotherapy: Theory and Practice.* New York: Harper and Row.

Pearlstein, Steven. 2016. Meet the Parents Who Won't Let Their Children Study Literature. *WashingtonPost.com.* https://www.washingtonpost.com/posteverything/wp/2016/09/02/meet-the-parents-who-wont-let-their-children-study-literature/?utm_term=68d0d86b3c3b. Accessed 1 Nov 2016.

Poe, Edgar Allan. 1899a. The Business Man (1940). In *Standard Edition of the Works of Edgar Allan Poe, Vol. II,* ed. John H. Ingram, pp. 560–569. London: A & C Black.

———. 1899b. The Man in the Crowd (1840). In *Standard Edition of the Works of Edgar Allan Poe, Vol. II,* ed. John H. Ingram, pp. 314–323. London: A & C Black.

———. 1899c. The Man That Was Used Up (1938). In *Standard Edition of the Works of Edgar Allan Poe, Vol. II,* ed. John H. Ingram, pp. 549–559. London: A & C Black.

———. 1899d. The Murders in the Rue Morgue (1841). In *Standard Edition of the Works of Edgar Allan Poe, Vol. I,* ed. John H. Ingram, pp. 404–441. London: A & C Black.

———. 1899e. The Philosophy of Composition (1841). In *Standard Edition of the Works of Edgar Allan Poe, Vol. III,* ed. John H. Ingram, pp. 266–278. London: A & C Black.

———. 1899f. The Purloined Letter (1844). In *Standard Edition of the Works of Edgar Allan Poe, Vol. I,* ed. John H. Ingram, pp. 494–513. London: A & C Black.

Pope, Rob. *1994. Textual Intervention: Critical and Creative Strategies for Literary Studies.* New York: Routledge.

Ramsay, Stephen. 2011a. *Reading Machines.* Chicago: University of Illinois Press.

———. 2011b. Who's In and Who's Out. *StephenRamsay.us.* http://stephenramsay.us/text/2011/01/08/whos-in-and-whos-out/. Accessed 1 November 2016.

———. 2012. Stanley and Me. *StephenRamsay.us.* http://stephenramsay.us/text/2012/11/08/stanley-and-me/. Accessed 1 November 2016.

Sample, Mark. 2011. The Digital Humanities Is Not About Building, It's About Sharing. *SampleReality.com.* http://www.samplereality.com/2011/05/25/the-digital-humanities-is-not-about-building-its-about-sharing/. Accessed 1 Nov 2016.

Samuels, Lisa, and Jerome McGann. 1999. Deformance and Interpretation. *New Literary History* 20 (1): 25–56.
Silverberg, William. 1948. The Concept of Transference. *The Psychoanalytic Quarterly* 17: 501–539.
Szasz, Thomas S. 1963. The Concept of Transference. *The International Journal of Psychoanalysis* 44: 432–443.
Thompson, Clara. 1945. Transference as a Therapeutic Instrument. *Interpersonal and Biological Processes* 8: 273–278.
———. 1956. The Role of the Analyst's Personality in Therapy. *American Journal of Psychotherapy* 10 (2): 347–367.

Index[1]

[1]Note: Page numbers followed by "n" refer to notes.

G. Basu Thakur, J.M. Dickstein (eds.), *Lacan and the Nonhuman*,
The Palgrave Lacan Series, DOI 10.1007/978-3-319-63817-1

Kolibri 360 GmbH
Ferdinand-Jühlke-Straße 7
99095 Erfurt, Deutschland
produktsicherheit@kolibri360.de